International Lifeguard Training Program™

Third Edition Revised

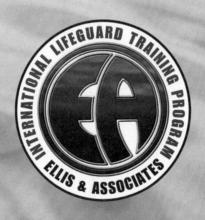

Ellis & Associates®

Latest CPR and ECC Guidelines

Jones and Bartlett Publishers
World Headquarters
40 Tall Pine Drive
Sudbury, MA 01776
www.jbpub.com
www.jblearning.com

Jones and Bartlett's books and products are available through most bookstores and online booksellers. To contact Jones and Bartlett Publishers directly, call 800-832-0034, fax 978-443-8000, or visit our website www.jbpub.com.

Substantial discounts on bulk quantities of Jones and Bartlett's publications are available to corporations, professional associations, and other qualified organizations. For details and specific discount information, contact the special sales department at Jones and Bartlett via the above contact information or send an email to specialsales@jbpub.com.

Production Credits

Chief Executive Officer: Clayton Jones
Chief Operating Officer: Donald W. Jones, Jr.
President, Higher Education and Professional Publishing:
  Robert Holland
V.P., Sales and Marketing: William J. Kane
V.P., Production and Design: Anne Spencer
V.P., Manufacturing and Inventory Control: Therese Connell
Executive Vice President, JB Learning: Larry Newell
Publisher, Public Safety: Kimberly Brophy
Managing Editor: Carol Guerrero

Associate Managing Editor: Robyn Schafer
Production Editor: Karen Ferreira
Photo Research Manager/Photographer: Kimberly Potvin
Director of Marketing: Alisha Weisman
Interior Design: Shepherd, Inc.
Cover Design: Anne Spencer
Composition: Shepherd, Inc.
Text Printing and Binding: Courier Kendallville
Cover Printing: Courier Kendallville
Cover photo © Jones and Bartlett Publishers, Inc.

The procedures and protocols in this book are based on the most current recommendations of responsible medical sources. Ellis & Associates and the Publisher, however, make no guarantee as to, and assume no responsibility for, the correctness, sufficiency, or completeness of such information or recommendations. Other or additional safety measures may be required under particular circumstances.

This textbook is intended solely as a guide to the appropriate procedures to be employed when rendering emergency care to pool, waterpark, and open water facility guests. It is not intended as a statement of standards of care required in any particular situation, because circumstances and the guest's physical condition can vary widely from one situation to another. Nor is it intended that this textbook shall in any way advise lifeguards concerning legal authority to perform the activities or procedures discussed. Such local determinations should be made only with the aid of legal counsel.

Some images in this book feature models. These models do not necessarily endorse, represent, or participate in the activities represented in the images.

To order this book please use ISBN 978-1-4496-2896-3

Library of Congress Cataloging-in-Publication Data

International lifeguard training program / Ellis & Associates.— 3rd ed.
   p. cm.
   Rev. ed. of: National pool and waterpark lifeguard training. 2nd ed.
   Includes bibliographical references and index.
   ISBN-13: 978-0-7637-4198-3 (alk. paper)
   ISBN-10: 0-7637-4198-1 (alk. paper)
   1. Lifeguards—Training of—Handbooks, manuals, etc. I. Ellis & Associates. II. National pool and waterpark lifeguard training.
   GV838.72.E45 2007
   797.2'10289—dc22   2006027170
   6048
Printed in the United States of America.
15 14   11

Contents

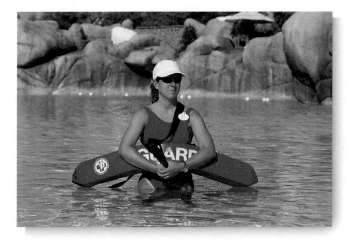

Part 1: Lifeguarding Responsibilities

Part 2: Responding to Emergencies

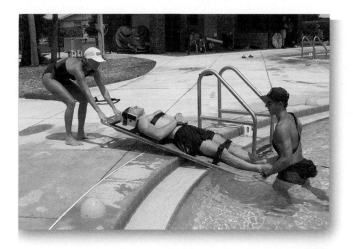

Part 3: Lifeguards as First Responders

Part 4: Open Water Lifeguarding

Preface

Congratulations on your decision to become an Ellis & Associates (E&A) licensed lifeguard or International Lifeguard Training Program™ (ILTP) Course Completion lifeguard. Following successful completion of the ILTP™, you will join a select group of aquatic professionals who apply proven state-of-the-art aquatic injury prevention practices in emergency incidents. As a result of E&A's emphasis on prevention, professionalism, and accountability, our safety record is unsurpassed in the aquatic industry.

HISTORY

Previously known as the National Pool and Waterpark Lifeguard Training Program™ (NPWLTP), the ILTP™ was originally developed in 1983 to address waterpark safety issues. Due to great demand for this quality program, it quickly expanded into pools, open water environments, and resorts. The new name, International Lifeguard Training Program™ (ILTP), reflects this expansion. Over its more than 20-year history, this training program has been credited by national and international agencies for revolutionizing the standards of the aquatic safety industry. The ILTP™/NPWLTP™ has led the industry in:

- Elevating professional lifeguard standards
- Using operational safety audits for lifeguard accountability
- Developing the 10/20 and 10/3 protection rules and proactive risk management standards including proactive bottom scanning and vigilance awareness training as the recognized standard of care
- Instituting body substance isolation (BSI) precautions to protect lifeguards from disease transmission
- Introducing the use of supplemental oxygen support, resuscitation masks, bag valve masks, manual suction devices, and automated external defibrillators (AEDs) to enhance resuscitation efforts
- Eliminating body contact rescues and advocating the exclusive use of the rescue tube
- Establishing a national database for injury prevention

- Incorporating distance education for both initial and refresher lifeguard training

THE E&A "MAKE IT WORK" PHILOSOPHY

Lifeguard rescue skills are best learned in the water, under the watchful eye of an E&A ILTP™ instructor. Once you have gained competency in these basic skills, you will apply what you have learned to real-life simulated incidents. This is where the ILTP™ objective-driven curriculum and E&A "make it work" philosophy become apparent.

The ILTP™ curriculum and philosophy stress that it is not as important to execute textbook-perfect rescues (which seldom occur in real life) as it is for lifeguards to solve problems and overcome adverse situations that might arise during a rescue effort. As long as the rescue is conducted effectively and techniques used provide maximum safety for both guests and lifeguards, then the rescue is a success. In this respect, the ILTP™ rescue philosophy differs significantly from that of other nationally recognized lifeguard training programs.

The ILTP™ emphasis is on effectively preventing aquatic emergencies by aggressively and proactively scanning zones, consistently monitoring guests, enforcing rules, and responding to emergencies effectively through lifeguard teamwork. Unlike other national lifeguard training programs, the ILTP™ focuses on team lifeguarding and "make it work" concepts rather than perfect individual rescue skills.

Another unique component of the ILTP™ is that lifeguard candidates learn to lifeguard while participating in class activities. In this way, they gain hands-on lifeguarding experience before they complete the course. ILTP™ is the only international lifeguard training program to mandate apprentice lifeguard experience in its training curriculum. The ILTP™ provides lifeguards with the knowledge and skills necessary to conduct themselves in the most professional manner and with confidence in their abilities.

Every aquatic facility is unique, and it is beyond the scope of this training manual and the ILTP™ to address all potential differences. To this end, ILTP™

lifeguards must rely on the management personnel at each individual aquatic facility to provide facility-specific information to supplement this training.

THE REAL JOB OF A LIFEGUARD

As a professional lifeguard, you will have two primary responsibilities:

- Preventing aquatic emergencies
- Conducting rescues and providing emergency care

If you believe lifeguarding is nothing more than a fun job with a chance to get a beautiful tan, you should think again. Lifeguarding is a glamorous job. Many lifeguards may be athletic, physically attractive, active, and young, and it is fair to say the position is highly regarded. Having a job with such high status could tempt you to concentrate on the wrong people and places while you are lifeguarding. If you let yourself become distracted by such other interests while you are supposed to be protecting guests in your facility, it could be the most tragic mistake you ever make. It is common for the glamour associated with lifeguarding to wear off quickly after you begin working, and you will discover what lifeguarding is truly about—preventing drowning.

If you decide to proceed with the ILTP™ course, successfully complete the training, and are employed as a lifeguard, it will undoubtedly become one of the most challenging and rewarding jobs you will ever experience.

Richard A. Carroll
Sr. VP/COO
Ellis & Associates

Acknowledgements

The task of writing, editing, reviewing, and producing a high quality training manual is complex. Many talented people have been involved in the original development of this manual. E&A is proud to be associated with so many dedicated professionals. To name everyone would be an impossible task, so we trust that they all recognize our sincere appreciation for their assistance by this notation. There are, however, several individuals, agencies, and organizations whose contributions to our program and publications over the years warrant special attention:

REVIEWERS AND EDITORS

Denise Beckson, Richard A. Carroll, Scott Deisley, Jeff Ellis, Franceen Gonzalez, Grant Goold, Ron Guest, Gary Henry, Jeff Henry, Haydn Holmes, Rob Klok, Joe Martinez, Luke Martinez, Dennis Mattey, Joseph Minninger, Larry Newell, Chris Perry, Louise Priest, Shannon Purtell, Randy Renstrom, Gary Reuter, Shelly Rucinski, Vera Solis, Joseph Stefanyak, Ron Sutula, Katie Timm, and Melissa Timmons.

AGENCIES AND ORGANIZATIONS

APEX Parks and Recreation, Atlantis-Bahamas, City of Portland, City of Tempe, College Station Parks and Recreation Department, Columbia Association, Dorney Park & Wildwater Kingdom, Jumeirah-International Dubai, Noah's Ark, Pointe South Mountain Resort, Rockford Park District, Schlitterbahn, Walt Disney World, YMCA Middle Tennessee, and all other E&A client facilities.

Introduction

COURSE OVERVIEW

Professional lifeguards prevent people from drowning. If lifeguards do not perform adequately, people may die.

Each year, ILTP™ lifeguards serve facilities that include waterparks, public pools, private pools, resorts, and open water environments (including ocean and bay fronts). ILTP™ lifeguards protect more than 100 million guests visiting these facilities and perform over 40,000 rescues annually. In many of these situations, if lifeguards had not intervened, guests would have drowned.

Ellis & Associates' International Lifeguard Training Program™ provides professional lifeguard training to protect guests and lifeguards from catastrophic injury and drowning. The purpose of the ILTP™ is to equip you with the skills and technical knowledge you need to become an effective member of your aquatic facility's emergency response team. An E&A License or ILTP™ Course Completion Card will show that you have participated in levels of training that exceed a reasonable standard. For waterpark and open water lifeguards, your training will include rescue techniques specifically designed for use in moving water.

The material in this textbook and related coursework will be taught by an approved E&A ILTP™ instructor. The International Lifeguard Training Program™ is divided into the following training courses:

- Shallow water lifeguard training
- Pool lifeguard training
- Special facilities lifeguard training

Skills you will learn in the ILTP™ course include:

- Anticipating how and where incidents will occur
- Recognizing incidents
- Effectively managing incidents
- Thinking critically about possible complications
- Acting in a professional manner
- Protecting your safety and the safety of others

You must be able to react and execute effective rescues without stopping to think about how to perform various parts of a skill. In addition to this course, regular in-service training sessions will help you build confidence and competence. During the course, you will learn how to manage situations by simulating real-life emergencies. You will learn skills that are safe, practical, and effective.

COURSE REQUIREMENTS

The following information outlines the various International Lifeguard Training Program™ course requirements and specifications.

1. Minimum Age to Obtain an E&A License or ILTP™ Course Completion Card
   - Shallow water lifeguard: 15 years of age
   - Pool lifeguard: 15 years of age
   - Special facilities lifeguard: 16 years of age

All certification is valid for one year.

2. Prerequisite Skills and Physical Requirements

Distance swim using crawl or breaststroke without resting:

- Shallow water lifeguard: 50 yards
- Pool lifeguard: 100 yards
- Special facilities lifeguard: 200 yards

Feet-first surface dive and retrieval of a 10-pound brick:

- Shallow water lifeguard: From a depth of 5 feet, and must be able to swim a distance of 10 feet under water
- Pool lifeguard: From a minimum depth of 8 feet (or deepest depth of facility)
- Special facilities lifeguard: From a minimum depth of 8 feet (or deepest depth of facility)

Treading water without using arms:

- Shallow water lifeguard: Not required
- Pool lifeguard: 1 minute
- Special facilities lifeguard: 2 minutes

Additional physical requirements:

- Lifeguards must be able to perform rescue skills in the working environment and must be able to demonstrate the ability to work efficiently within the parameters of an established Emergency Action Plan (EAP). Lifeguards must be able to exit from a pool at any point without the use of ladders, steps, or a zero-depth exit. (ANSI D-1 wave pools and pools with a similar distance from the static water line to the deck would be exempt from this requirement.)

- Participating in the ILTP™ requires that lifeguard candidates be in good physical condition. Any limitations that may present a health or safety hazard while participating in training or while on duty should be communicated to the facility/instructor. Employer may have additional physical or health requirements in order to be employed. These limitations may require additional assistance that will need to be provided by the employer.

3. Facilities Where Certification Is Valid

- Shallow water lifeguard: Any facility where water depth is 5 feet or less (excluding open water environments)
- Pool lifeguard: Any facility where water depth is not greater than 16 feet (excluding open water environments)
- Special facility lifeguard: Any facility where the pool depth is greater than 5 feet and/or there are wave pools or open water environments

4. Qualifications for E&A License or ILTP™ Course Completion Card

- Meet all course prerequisites
- Attend all class periods
- Execute all rescue skills and all First Aid, CPR, and AED skills to "test ready" levels
- Pass all written and water practical examinations (80 percent or better)

5. Course Rules

- Be on time for all sessions.
- Protect yourself from the sun (including hat, sunglasses, and sunscreen when outdoors).
- Enter the water feet first at all times.
- Lifeguard must be on duty at all times when a class is in the water.
- When using a rescue tube, keep it between the guest and yourself.
- Exhibit professionalism and maturity at all times.

6. General Course Information

- All courses include lifeguard first aid and Healthcare provider BLS skills for adults, children, and infants, as well as oxygen administration skills and automated external defibrillator (AED) training.
- If you do not pass all the requirements for any class you are taking, you must repeat the entire course to be eligible for an E&A License or ILTP™ Course Completion Card.

7. E&A License or ILTP™ Course Completion Card Validity and Suspension

Licenses and Course Completion Cards are valid only when you:

- Meet all course prerequisites
- Pass all written (80 percent or better) and water practical examinations
- Demonstrate proper attitude, maturity, and judgment
- Complete site-specific facility training

Your E&A License may be suspended or revoked for cause at any time; read the license agreement carefully to be sure you understand your responsibilities. ILTP™ Course Completion Cards are not subject to suspension terms or conditions.

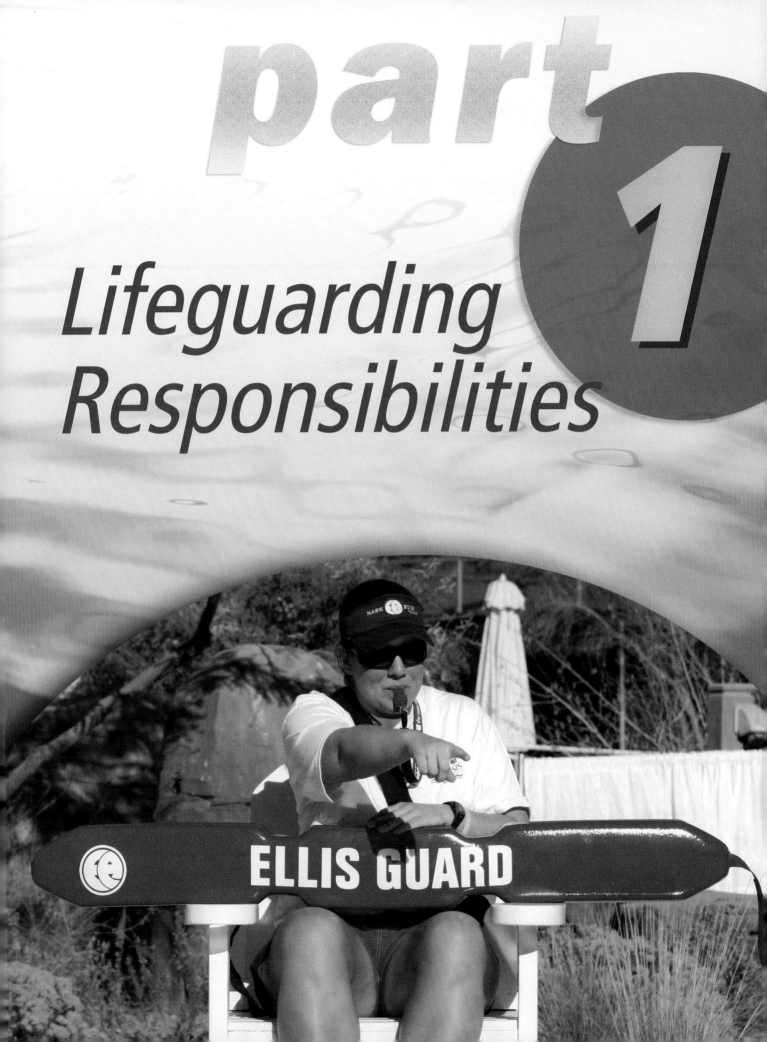

part 1

Lifeguarding Responsibilities

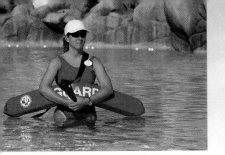

Lifeguard Accountability and Professionalism

INTRODUCTION

The International Lifeguard Training Program™ (ILTP) teaches you how to act and respond as a professional lifeguard. You will learn how to anticipate, recognize, and manage an aquatic emergency. You are the critical, frontline component of a professional water safety and **risk management** system at an aquatic facility.

Lifeguards are required to perform in accordance with practices that comprise a **standard of care**. A general definition of the standard of care is the degree of care a responsible person would take to prevent an injury to another person. The standard of care expected of lifeguards who complete the ILTP™ consists of:

- Proactive swimmer protection that meets the 10/20 protection standard
- "Test-ready" skill maintenance
- Demonstration of a professional image

Each of these concepts is described in detail in later sections.

ACCOUNTABILITY

The job of a lifeguard is more demanding than most people realize. You are responsible for the lives of many guests on a daily basis. As an ILTP™ lifeguard, you must be willing to accept the responsibility and accountability that go along with the job. This means that you must look and behave like a professional at all times when you are working; how you conduct yourself when you are not working also reflects on your professionalism.

You must maintain your personal skills and knowledge at a "test-ready" level. Whether your job is part-time, seasonal, or full-time, you will be judged as a professional—one who is able to provide the standard of care required (**Figure 1.1**).

As a professional lifeguard, you are accountable to:

- *The guests using your facility*—You are expected to provide a safe environment for the guests, minimizing hazardous situations whenever possible and responding appropriately to emergency situations.
- *Your employer*—You will be expected to perform the duties of your job, established by your organization. You must be dedicated to your job and

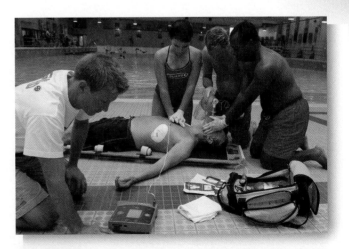

FIG 1.1 Lifeguards are always expected to provide a proper standard of care for guests.

perform at or above your employer's expectations. While at work, you will be evaluated as a professional lifeguard on a daily basis by the guests and your employer.

- *Yourself*—Confidence is a key characteristic of a successful lifeguard. You have to believe in yourself and understand that you are responsible for human lives. You must know all of the responsibilities of your position and maintain your knowledge and skill levels. You must recognize, respond to, and manage aquatic emergencies quickly and effectively. You should evaluate yourself on a continuous basis. Ask yourself: "Am I the type of person with whom I would entrust the lives of my family?"

MAINTAINING A PROFESSIONAL IMAGE

As a lifeguard, you will need to demonstrate a **professional image**. You are part of your facility's team, contributing to the total operation of the facility and protection of the guests. If you look and act like a professional, the facility looks like a professionally-run facility (**Figure 1.2**). If guests view you as a professional, they will respond to your requests because they believe in you. If guests have no respect for you or your position, they will disregard your requests, which will have a dramatic effect during an emergency situation.

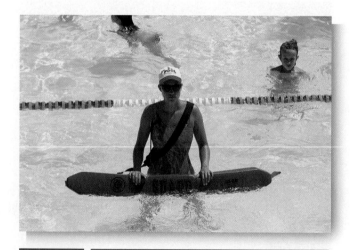

FIG 1.2   A lifeguard must look professional and be easily identified by guests.

You can present a professional image by being:

- *Punctual*—Arrive at work ahead of time.
- *In proper uniform*—Look neat, clean, and easily identifiable as a lifeguard.
- *Prepared*—Have the items you need to do the job (whistle, hydration, sun protection, etc.).
- *Pleasant*—Act cordially to guests and coworkers at all times; smile.
- *Attentive*—Keep your eyes on the zone of protection (see Chapter 2) and avoid distractions.
- *Vigilant*—Maintain your lifeguarding skills at peak performance level (test-ready).
- *Knowledgeable*—Know and enforce the facility rules.

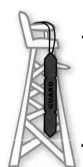

tips from the top

Guests will respect you and respond to your requests if you act professionally.

ELLIS & ASSOCIATES CLIENT FACILITY AUDITS

ILTP™ lifeguards who are not employed at E&A client facilities are not subject to E&A Aquatic Safety Operational Audits. However, E&A licensed lifeguards who perform duties at an E&A facility will participate in Aquatic Safety Operational Audits, which are a major component of the E&A Comprehensive Aquatic Risk Management Program. During these **audits**, Ellis & Associates staff will visit facilities unannounced to observe lifeguards and the normal day-to-day operation of the facility. You will be evaluated on four aspects of your job:

1. Your professionalism and on-the-stand performance
2. Your ability to remain vigilant and effectively meet the swimmer protection standards
3. Your level of rescue readiness
4. Your ability to protect yourself from the environment

The purpose of the E&A audit is (1) to identify potential aquatic risk exposures before they become catastrophic and (2) to increase the awareness, education, and implementation of effective aquatic risk management principles to eliminate or reduce those risk exposures. It is not the intent of the auditor to catch you or your facility doing something wrong. Overall, the auditor will evaluate you and your team's ability to anticipate, recognize, and manage an aquatic emergency.

The Aquatic Safety Operational Audit is a risk management tool utilized by E&A client facilities to identify and address potential risk exposures before they become serious problems. Subsequent audits will validate the reduction or elimination of previously identified risk exposures, and this information will become part of the facility's risk management documentation. Professional lifeguards perform well during audits because they are always attentive and committed to preventing, recognizing, and managing aquatic emergencies (**Figure 1.3**).

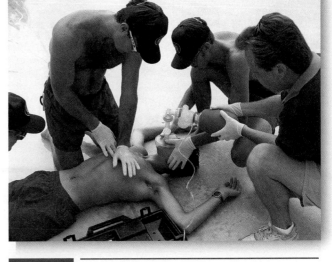

FIG 1.3 You may be asked to demonstrate rescue skills during an audit.

WRAP-UP

Being a professional lifeguard involves:

- Being prepared physically and mentally for your job
- Practicing your skills
- Recognizing that you are accountable for your actions
- Acting responsibly
- Being committed to doing your job well

WHAT YOU SHOULD HAVE LEARNED

After reading this chapter and completing the related course work, you should be able to:

1. Identify to whom lifeguards are accountable while performing their job.
2. Identify ways to project a professional image as a lifeguard.

CHAPTER 1 Lifeguard Skills

AUDIT PERFORMANCE

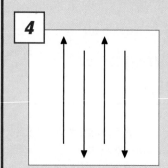

Sun Protection
Sunglasses, hydration, and shade.

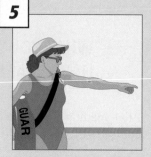

Rescue Tube
Hold the tube professionally; gather strap.

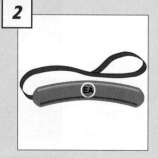

Posture
Alert; anticipatory.

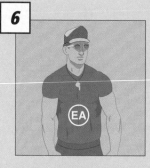

Scanning
Know your zone; have a scanning pattern. Use the 10/20 protection standard (see Chapter 2).

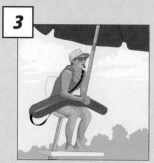

Communication
Assertive, respective; use whistle and hand signals (see Chapter 3).

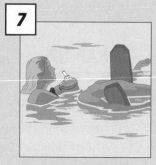

Professionalism and Uniform
Positive image; easily recognizable.

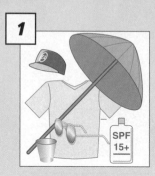

Rescue Skills
Frequent in-service training; always be "test-ready."

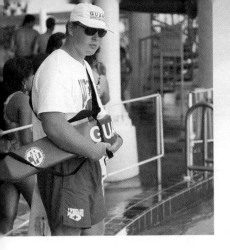

Awareness and Recognition

INTRODUCTION

Consider how you will actually spend your time as a lifeguard. You will not always be making rescues and caring for distressed guests. Instead, most of your time will be spent preventing potentially hazardous situations and protecting the guests at your facility.

PROTECTING GUESTS

The International Lifeguard Training Program™ uses an approach known as the **10/20 protection standard** as a guiding principle for aquatic facility safety. This approach means that while scanning an area, the lifeguard has 10 seconds to recognize that a guest is in **distress** and an additional 20 seconds to reach the guest and begin rendering aid (**Figure 2.1**). Recognition, reaction, and management of a guest in distress within the first 30 seconds has proven to effectively save lives and has resulted in more successful out-

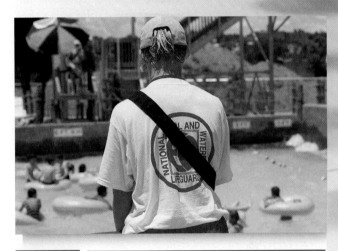

FIG 2.1 The 10/20 protection standard can help you be prepared for any situation.

comes. By using the 10/20 protection standard rule, facilities can better determine the appropriate position for lifeguard stations and the size of each zone of protection.

tips from the top

The 10/20 protection standard provides 10 seconds to recognize a guest is in distress and an additional 20 seconds to reach the guest and begin rendering aid.

Zones of Protection

Each lifeguard station or position is assigned a specific area of responsibility, commonly called a **zone of protection**. In a facility with multiple lifeguards and zones, zones may change when staffing is modified. As a lifeguard, you must be able to clearly see every part of your assigned zone. In order to do this you must:

- Clearly understand the parameters of your zone of protection.

- Stay focused, not allowing yourself to become distracted.
- Continually scan the entire zone (top, middle, and bottom of the water), moving both your head and your eyes.
- Be able to reach the farthest part of your zone within 20 seconds.
- Identify problem areas and take corrective measures to meet the standard of care before guests begin using the area.

Every facility should have a chart showing the zone(s) for each lifeguard position (**Figure 2.2a-c**). Depending on the number of guests and unique features of the facility, these zones may need to be adjusted. As a lifeguard, it is your responsibility to know the exact area for which you are accountable at any given station. This means you could be responsible for several different zones depending on the station, pool design, or number of guests. Zones should overlap to be certain that no area is left unprotected. If lifeguard stations are eliminated (as they sometimes are when there are fewer guests), lifeguard positions and zones of protection may be adjusted. Always know your zone of protection; you are accountable. If you do not know your zone of protection, then ask a supervisor before assuming responsibility for that area of the facility.

Vigilance

Vigilance means constant and careful attention to your zone(s) of protection. You must avoid being distracted when scanning your zone(s). Guarding the water may become routine or even boring, but you must stay alert at all times, because guests may enter your zone at any moment. Do not compromise the safety of the guests—no matter what the circumstances. It only takes a second for a person to slip under the water.

Proactive Scanning

As you vigilantly watch your zone, your head and eyes need to move in regular patterns. This movement is known as **scanning**. There are several scanning patterns that are commonly used by lifeguards (**Figure 2.3a–f**). You will need to develop a scanning pattern that works for you. You may find that changing your scanning pattern occasionally helps you maintain vigilance.

   The shape of your zone is not important. It may be a rectangle or a semicircle, or it may be defined by the

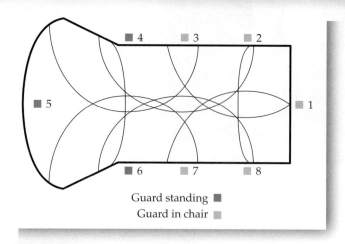

Guard standing ■
Guard in chair ■

FIG 2.2a Lifeguard zone coverage.

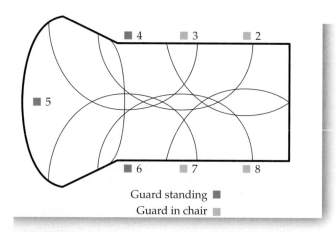

Guard standing ■
Guard in chair ■

FIG 2.2b Lifeguard zone coverage with no lifeguard in position 1.

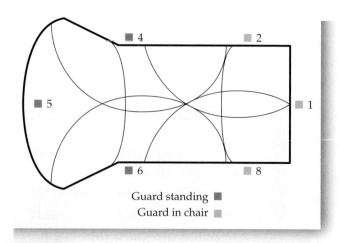

Guard standing ■
Guard in chair ■

FIG 2.2c Lifeguard zone coverage with no lifeguards in positions 3 and 7.

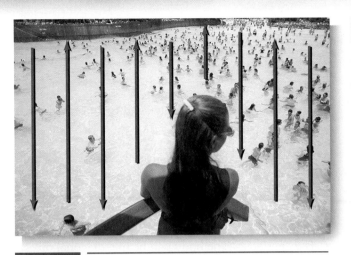

FIG 2.3a Up and down scanning pattern.

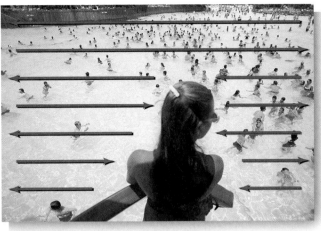

FIG 2.3b Side to side scanning pattern.

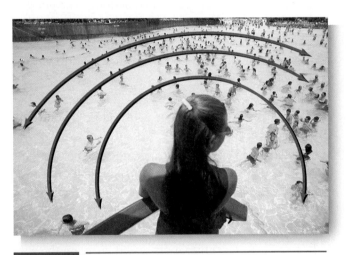

FIG 2.3c Circular scanning pattern.

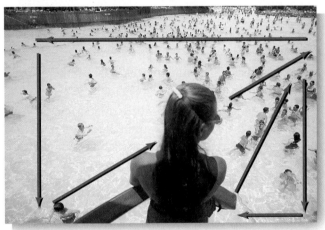

FIG 2.3d Double triangle scanning pattern.

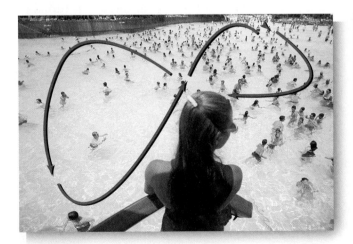

FIG 2.3e Figure eight scanning pattern.

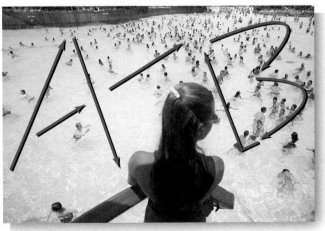

FIG 2.3f Alphabet scanning pattern.

shape of your facility. Each zone will have its own unique scanning challenges.

A scan of the zone should be completed within a time frame that quickly allows you to recognize that someone is in distress and react to the situation. If you have a concern about your ability to maintain the 10/20 protection standard, discuss it with your supervisor immediately.

With experience, you will develop your own scanning technique. Here are some suggestions to help you scan more effectively:

- Know the exact zone to be scanned and develop a scanning pattern that covers all of it.
- Know where your zone overlaps with another lifeguard's zone.
- Check your entire zone each time you scan, regardless of guest concentration.
- Know **high risk** areas. You may need more time to scan these areas.
- When replacing another lifeguard, ask if there are any special circumstances you should know about.
- Remember that the pool is three dimensional—view the surface, middle, and bottom of the water. If there is glare on the surface restricting your ability to see underwater, change your position so that you can see the entire zone from all three dimensions. Communicate to management every time you experience an environmental issue that reduces your ability to view all three dimensions of the zone.
- Periodically check the lifeguard who would back you up and the lifeguard who you would back up.
- Scan directly beneath your stand and to the extremes of your zone.
- Be active and use the 5-minute strategy—sit, stand, stroll, and change posture, position, or perspective every 5 minutes to remain alert and active.
- Maintain good posture. It helps to stay alert and maintain a professional appearance.

You may need to continually adjust your scanning pattern to accommodate certain situations in your zone. For example, you may have several different groups of guests with varying swimming abilities in your zone. You may need to pause a little longer on certain individuals in those areas. Remember, if glare or shadows on the surface prevent you from viewing your zone, change position so that you can see the entire zone and communicate the issue to your supervisor immediately.

RECOGNIZING A GUEST IN DISTRESS

A guest in distress in the water will be in one of three locations:

1. On the surface
2. Below the surface, within arm's reach
3. Below the surface, beyond arm's reach

Signs of a guest in distress include (**Figure 2.4**):

- *Body position*—The body will be in a diagonal or vertical position. Legs are not kicking and arms are extended out to the side. It may look like the guest is trying to reach or grab for something. The guest may have turned toward safety (a lifeguard, a wall, or a lane line).
- *Movement*—There will be little or no forward movement.
- *Appearance*—All effort is expended to stay above the water. Eyes may be open or tightly closed. Long hair may cover the face.
- *Breathing*—In an attempt to breathe, the head will usually be held back to keep the mouth above the surface of the water. The guest is attempting to concentrate only on breathing while on the surface. There may be little or no calling out for help.

It is easier to recognize a distressed guest on the surface than underwater. Even in a clear pool, it may be difficult to recognize a distressed guest who is submerged. The number of guests in the water, turbidity

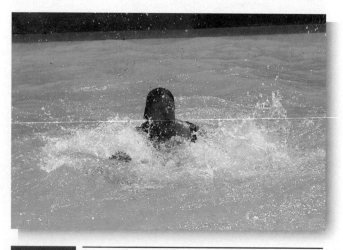

FIG 2.4   A guest in distress on the surface.

(murkiness of the water), or glare can make it almost impossible to see under the surface. When this happens, you will need to put yourself in a position to see your entire zone. If you cannot, alert your supervisor about the problem immediately.

A guest on the bottom of a pool may look like a blurred spot. When water clarity and crowd conditions allow, guard from the bottom of the pool up. If you notice anything on the bottom of a pool and cannot identify it, GO! (**Figure 2.5**)

Any lack of movement demands your immediate attention, quick evaluation, and appropriate response. The faster you recognize a guest in distress, the more effective you will be in handling the incident. Be proactive; it is better to immediately respond and rescue a guest who looks distressed than to wait until he or she is really in trouble. Remember, as a professional lifeguard, you must maintain the 10/20 protection standard and recognize a guest in distress within 10 seconds.

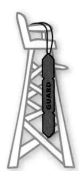

tips from the top

Lifeguard from the bottom up: If you don't know, GO!

DROWNING

An understanding of the **drowning** process will help you recognize a guest who needs immediate rescue. A guest who is drowning can be either active or passive. **Active drowning** victims may struggle on the surface for a short period before submerging. **Passive (silent) drowning** victims can slip quickly and silently beneath the surface. Passive drowning victims do not struggle on the surface, and lifeguards are given no warning signs. Passive drowning can be caused by various physical conditions or situations, such as heart attack, shallow water blackout, head injury, seizure, stroke, or reaction to alcohol or drugs.

The time span for the complete drowning process can vary from seconds to minutes. Children seem to move through the drowning process more quickly than adults. A child may appear to be bobbing in the water. This behavior may actually be an attempt to get to the surface. The pattern of distress for children may include a brief struggle once completely submerged, followed quickly by unconsciousness (**Figure 2.6**). The different stages of drowning are described in **Table 2.1**.

Death by Drowning

When a guest is drowning, breathing and circulation cease, and the guest enters cardiac arrest. The heart does not pump blood throughout the body, and vital organs do not receive oxygen-rich blood.

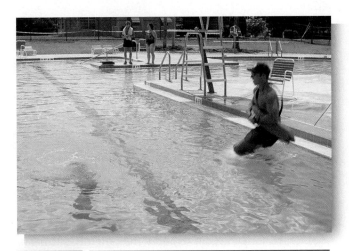

FIG 2.5 A submerged guest may be difficult to see.

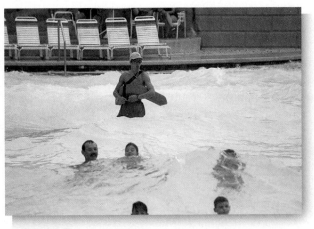

FIG 2.6 An inexperienced swimmer in water over his or her head could panic and quickly become a drowning victim.

TABLE 2.1 *The Drowning Process*

Stage	Description	What to Look For
Surprise	The guest recognizes the danger and is afraid.	• Vertical or diagonal body position • Arms at or near the surface making random grasping or flapping motions • Little or no leg movement • Head tilted back, with face upward • Usually not making any sounds (more concerned with getting air than with calling for help)
Involuntary breath holding	Water enters the mouth, causing the epiglottis to close over the airway, which leads to suffocation.	• May continue to struggle • Usually no sounds • No breathing
Unconsciousness	Lack of breathing leads to loss of consciousness.	• No arm or leg movement • May sink to the bottom, either slowly or rapidly, or remain afloat (depends on factors such as body composition and residual air in the lungs)
Hypoxic convulsions	Lack of oxygen to the brain can lead to convulsions (seizure).	• Body rigidity • Jerking actions • Frothing at the mouth • Skin, especially the lips and face, turning pale, blue, or gray
Clinical death	Breathing and circulation stop; guest begins cardiac arrest.	• Unconsciousness • No pulse or breathing • No movement • Pale, blue, or grayish skin • Dilated pupils

If the guest has been without oxygen for only a few minutes and you provide immediate care, including cardiopulmonary resuscitation (CPR) and use of an automated external defibrillator (AED) (see Chapter 7), there is a chance that the guest may recover without permanent brain damage. The longer the guest is without adequate oxygen and circulation, the poorer the chance of recovery. Even if your care efforts are successful at the scene, many drowning victims die at the hospital as a result of secondary complications. Drowning guests need advanced life support as quickly as possible, so it is essential to activate your facility's emergency action plan (see Chapter 3) to summon EMS personnel immediately.

Types of Drowning

There are two types of drowning: wet and dry. These categories are based on whether water is present in the lungs following death. Eighty percent of drownings are

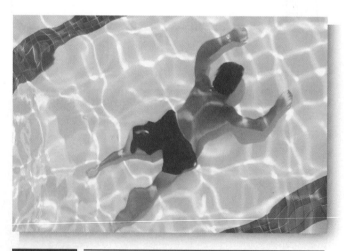

FIG 2.7   Submerged victims often result in wet drowning.

wet drownings, which occur when a person has been submerged long enough to allow the **epiglottis** to relax due to lack of oxygen. If the submerged person takes a spontaneous (agonal) breath, water enters the trachea and lungs, which results in wet drowning (**Figure 2.7**).

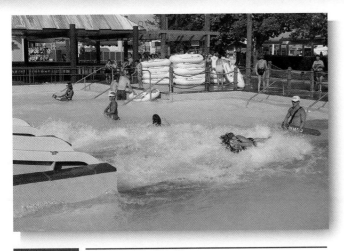

| **FIG 2.8** | High velocity activities, such as water slides, have the potential for dry drowning. |

Dry drowning, or asphyxiation, occurs when water makes contact with the epiglottis, causing it to spasm and close over the airway. This prevents air and water from entering the trachea and lungs, suffocating the drowning victim. Dry drowning is more likely to occur around speed slides, diving boards, or slides that end in a free-fall **(Figure 2.8)**.

SPECIAL CONCERNS

Certain situations allow you to anticipate potential incidents before they occur, including:

- Guests with a greater potential for becoming distressed
- Locations where guests are most likely to become distressed
- Certain days and times that statistically have high rescue rates

These situations are outlined in detail in **Table 2.2**.

WRAP-UP

Being a professional lifeguard involves:

- Maintaining the 10/20 protection standard
- Remaining vigilant at all times
- Understanding your zone of protection
- Knowing and using proactive scanning patterns
- Scanning your zone from the bottom up
- Recognizing special guests, locations, and times that are more likely to require rescues

TABLE 2.2 Special Concerns

Special Guests	Locations	Days/Times
Guests with greater potential for becoming distressed: • Children between the ages of 7 and 12 • Young children attended to by parents • Shorter individuals who may wade into deep water • People who cannot swim • Intoxicated guests • Guests with unusual or extreme body proportions • Elderly guests • Disabled guests • Guests not dressed in swimming attire • Guests wearing lifejackets	Attractions with a higher number of rescues: • Deep water • Wave pools (especially at the point where the waves break) • Activity pools • Slide catch pools • Hydraulic currents • Drop-off areas • Diving wells • Pool exits • Lake areas (especially areas beyond those designated for swimming)	Days and times when a higher number of rescues occur: • Mid-day (12–4 P.M.) • Holidays • Extremely hot days

≋ WHAT YOU SHOULD HAVE LEARNED

After reading this chapter and completing the related course work, you should be able to:

1. Explain and implement the 10/20 protection standard.

2. Explain the importance of vigilance while scanning.

3. Demonstrate proper scanning techniques.

4. Describe the different behavior patterns of a guest in distress.

5. Explain the phases of the drowning process.

6. Describe the different types of drowning.

7. Describe special situations in which lifeguards should be able to anticipate potential incidents before they occur.

CHAPTER 2 Lifeguard Skills

SCANNING

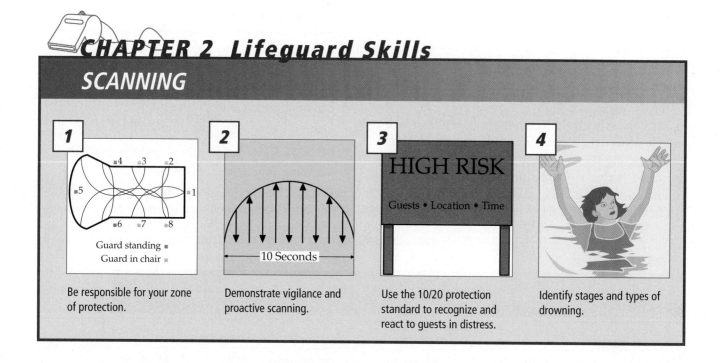

1 Be responsible for your zone of protection.

2 Demonstrate vigilance and proactive scanning.

3 Use the 10/20 protection standard to recognize and react to guests in distress.

4 Identify stages and types of drowning.

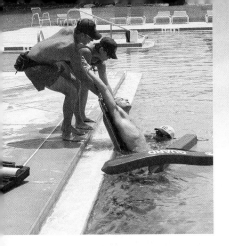

Reacting to an Emergency

〜 INTRODUCTION

In an emergency situation, people often become confused and excited; they may react without thinking. In doing so, they put themselves and others at even greater risk than the situation warrants. It isn't something people do on purpose; it just happens because there is no plan of action. Therefore, it is important for every facility to have an official **emergency action plan (EAP)** so that lifeguards and other staff members, known as **supplemental responders**, can respond effectively to emergencies. Supplemental responders are trained to provide rescue and patient care skills as part of the lifeguard team in accordance with the facility's EAP. At a minimum they must be capable of providing cardiopulmonary resuscitation (CPR); they must be able to use an automated external defibrillator (AED); and they must know deck extrication skills for both unconscious and suspected neck and back injury guests. Supplemental responders should be trained, staffed, scheduled and in-serviced to act as a "lifeguard," from an on-deck perspective.

In situations where there are no additional staff members on-site to assist a single lifeguard on duty, the need to include patrons and bystanders in the EAP may exist. The use of patrons and bystanders at single-guarded facilities presents many challenges and may not allow for effective emergency response or patient care and treatment. In these cases, the use of supplemental responders is recommended.

〜 EMERGENCY ACTION PLAN (EAP)

As a professional lifeguard, you cannot become confused or excited during an emergency; you must be in control of your actions and know what must be done. You cannot expose any guests or yourself to greater risk; your job is to minimize risk and prevent any further injury. To do your job effectively, you must have a plan of action. Every aquatic facility has an emergency action plan (EAP) that outlines a chain of events that will help you, your fellow lifeguards, and supplemental responders manage a wide range of emergency situations in the best manner possible (**Figure 3.1**).

Your facility will have a written plan outlining its EAP, which will be specifically designed for your location. You will need to read, discuss, and practice the plan, which covers common types of emergencies. In single lifeguard facilities, it is essential that the plan is communicated to, and practiced with, all supplemental responders who are part of the EAP. Sample emergency action plans can be found in Appendix A.

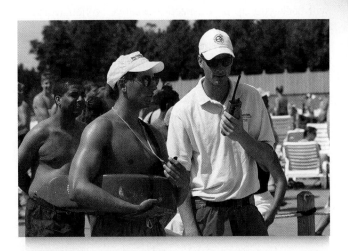

FIG 3.1 You need to be thoroughly familiar with your facility's emergency action plan to effectively manage an emergency.

An EAP outlines what should happen during an emergency. It begins with the recognition of the emergency and addresses actions such as the lifeguard's reaction, rescue, and care that should be provided to the guest. The plan should also include the actions supplemental responders must take to assist the lifeguard(s) with effecting the rescue, ensuring the safety of the remaining guests in the area, and providing for the transfer of care to **emergency medical services (EMS)** personnel. The plan also outlines the need to gather information about the emergency, such as witness statements and incident reports, as well as critiques and follow-up meetings.

The number of steps in an EAP will depend on the size of the facility and the number of staff available. Every facility will operate differently. No matter how large or small the aquatic facility may be, the most important part of any EAP is the lifeguard. If the lifeguard fails to recognize the emergency or fails to activate the EAP, the rest of the plan will fail.

Lifeguards usually activate the EAP by blowing their whistle. This alerts other lifeguards and supplemental responders that they are responding to an emergency and may need assistance. Even if they do not need help with the actual rescue, the guests in their zones will need to be supervised during the rescue.

Zone Coverage When the EAP Is Activated

The EAP must be set up to ensure that your Zone of Protection area will be covered while you assist a guest and that another lifeguard or supplemental responder will back you up if you need assistance. When working in a facility that has two or more lifeguards on duty at the time of the incident, the lifeguard to your left will usually assume responsibility for your Zone of Protection area if you leave your position during an emergency or need assistance. This also means that you are the backup for the lifeguard to your right. If you are the only lifeguard at the facility, your Zone of Protection area should be the entire pool. Lifeguard Zone of Protection areas should be defined to allow the lifeguard to view the entire Zone of Protection area including the surface, middle (subsurface), and bottom from the lifeguard position.

When you hear a whistle signaling an emergency, you should immediately check the lifeguard to your right. If that lifeguard has left the stand to assist a guest, you now have to expand your scanning pattern to cover both zones and to keep an eye on the lifeguard performing the rescue. Watch and be ready to assist that lifeguard if help is requested.

If you are in a stand and there is no lifeguard stand to your left, you can use one of these methods to handle this situation:

- The lifeguard to your right covers your zone and is your backup.
- Depending on the size of the facility and shape of the pool, the lifeguard across the pool will cover your zone and be your backup.

The specific procedure you use will be determined by your facility management.

When two or more lifeguards are required to leave their stations to perform a rescue, the "guard to your left" rule may not work. The zones may be too large for the remaining lifeguards to cover. If this is the situation, the attraction/facility must be closed and all guests cleared from the water. Once the emergency has passed and the lifeguards have returned to their stands, the attraction/facility can be reopened.

If there are enough lifeguards to safely cover all zones or replace guards who have entered the water, the attraction/facility may remain open. The EAP should provide for other lifeguards who may be on break to cover the Zone of Protection areas of the lifeguards involved in the rescue.

In facilities with only one or two lifeguards, the EAP must involve other staff (supplemental responders) who can clear the water and control the crowd. The supplemental responders must immediately clear the water of any and all swimmers so that no one is left in the water without lifeguard supervision. The EAP should clearly identify who is responsible for providing secondary response assistance and for clearing the Zone of Protection area while the rescue takes place. Supplemental responders must also be trained to assist with the rescue once the guest is on the pool deck and to provide emergency care or skills.

SAFETY PRECAUTIONS

When caring for a guest, always take preliminary steps to ensure your safety.

Scene Safety

Always assess the situation by conducting a scene safety survey before assisting a distressed guest. Scan the entire area to determine if any hazards are present, including sharp objects, dangerous environmental conditions, or hazardous materials. Make sure to account for these hazards and ensure your safety *before* responding.

Body Substance Isolation (BSI)

The most common hazards with which you will come into contact as a lifeguard are biological—infectious diseases that may be transmitted by contact with bodily fluids. **Body substance isolation (BSI)** safety precautions help prevent exposure to bodily fluids to ensure your safety. Always follow these precautions before treating an injured or distressed guest:

- Wear gloves before contacting an injured guest.
- Use protective equipment to guard your eyes and mouth.
- Dispose of needles and other sharp materials properly.
- Wash hands immediately after properly removing gloves.
- Clean hands and other areas that may have been exposed to bodily fluids.

COMMUNICATION

In an aquatic facility, communication can be difficult because of crowd noise, weather, acoustics, or distance. You must be able to communicate with guests to enforce rules, as well as with other lifeguards and supervisors. Whistles and hand signals are good ways to communicate around water and to overcome ambient noise. Many facilities also use telephones, two-way radios, megaphones, or other communication devices.

The following sections provide examples of ways to communicate in order to control your area and be able to notify other lifeguards or supervisors in different situations. Your facility may use these common signals or develop its own communication system. You need to know and practice the communication signals used in your facility.

Whistles

Your whistle will be your most frequently used piece of safety equipment. You will be required to have a whistle with you at all times when you are on duty. Your whistle should be in good working order, with a shrill tone that cuts through crowd noise. When you have to use your whistle, you should blow it loudly and firmly. You should have regular whistle-blowing practice. This teaches you to blow the whistle properly and helps you recognize its sound over crowd noise and other distractions. A few common whistle commands are:

- *One short whistle blast*—Get attention of guest(s)
- *Two short whistle blasts*—Get attention of lifeguard(s)
- *One long whistle blast*—Activate the EAP
- *Two long whistle blasts*—Indicate a major emergency

Hand Signals

Hand signals are primarily used with whistles to help communicate. When possible, you should hold the hand signal for 5 seconds to make sure it is noticed. A few common hand signals are:

- *Pointing*—Point to give direction. Pointing can be used with a whistle blast to indicate to guests what you would like them to do. This is also helpful when you would like to point out a certain guest to another lifeguard or supervisor (**Figure 3.2**).
- *Raised clenched fist*—This means that you need help. If you are on the deck, at the side of the pool, or in your stand, this may be used with whistle blasts. If you are in the water, you may not be able to use your whistle (**Figure 3.3**).

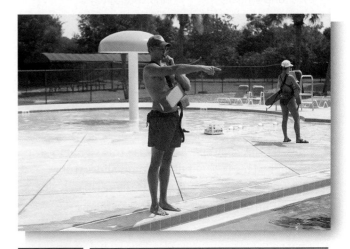

FIG 3.2 Blow your whistle loudly and firmly while pointing to get the attention of guests, other lifeguards, or supervisors.

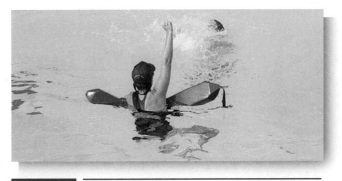

FIG 3.3 Lifeguard requesting assistance during a rescue.

TABLE 3.1 *Communication Signals*

Signal	Purpose	Action
One short whistle blast	Get the attention of a guest	After you get the guest's attention, it is best to use basic hand signals and speak clearly if you need to give further instructions. Avoid allowing frustration to turn your short whistle blast into a long one. A megaphone helps when you have to talk to a guest in a crowded facility.
Two short whistle blasts	Get the attention of another lifeguard or supervisor	As you blow your whistle, raise your hand or tap the top of your head. This lets the other lifeguards or supervisor know who has whistled and what is needed.
One long whistle blast	Activate the EAP	This indicates that you are leaving your stand to perform a rescue, someone has to cover your zone, and additional personnel may be needed. Wherever you are working, you should point to where you are going. In a wave pool you should hit the emergency stop button (E-stop), when present, to stop the waves. The lifeguard assigned by your facility's backup coverage plan will watch your zone in addition to his or her own. A head lifeguard or supervisor should respond to all emergencies whenever possible or practical.
Two long whistle blasts	Indicate a major emergency	This indicates a life-threatening situation. Additional lifeguards or personnel may be needed. The facility may need to be closed immediately and guests cleared from the area. Other lifeguards who are not involved in the rescue are responsible for securing the facility before providing additional support.

- *Crossed arms above the head*—Use this signal to stop dispatch. This is generally used on slides, tube rides, or other water attractions that dispatch riders.
- *Thumbs up*—This indicates it is all right to resume the activity.
- *Tapping the top of your head*—This signal means "Watch my area."

See **Table 3.1** for examples of how hand and whistle signals are used together to communicate in an aquatic facility.

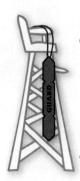

tips from the top

Two important emergency numbers are 9-1-1 to activate the EMS system and 800-222-1222 for Poison Control.

Other Communication Devices

In addition to whistles and hand signals, the following communication devices are used at aquatic facilities (**Figure 3.4**):

- *Megaphones*—These are especially useful in large or crowded facilities.
- *Telephones*—Telephones must be available for emergencies. The telephone numbers for emergency services must be posted near the telephone and be clearly visible. These phones must be used only for official business or emergencies.
- *Two-way radios*—These are used primarily among supervisors and medical staff.
- *Public address systems*—Announcements including emergency information can be communicated to your entire facility very quickly.

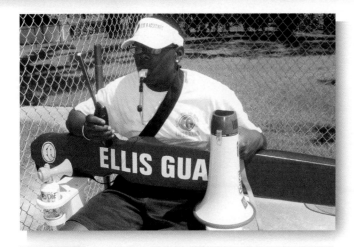

FIG 3.4   Devices used for communication.

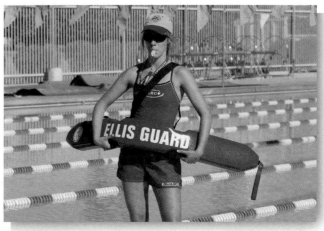

FIG 3.5   Rescue tubes provide excellent flotation during water emergencies.

TEAM LIFEGUARDING

No matter the size of the aquatic facility or the number of lifeguards on duty at any time, as a professional lifeguard, you are a member of an emergency response team. Once you activate the EAP, your signal is meant to draw together other lifeguards and support personnel. This is your team. They may cover your Zone of Protection area or provide other forms of assistance.

All team members must know their responsibilities during an emergency. The ultimate goal is to prevent drowning. The more each staff member can be part of the team process, the more effective the EAP will be.

RESCUES AND ASSISTS

An **assist** occurs when you help a guest, either from the deck or in the water, and you are still able to maintain zone coverage within the 10/20 protection standard. A **rescue** occurs when a guest would not be able to get to the pool surface or deck without lifeguard intervention. It applies to any situation for which the EAP is activated.

RESCUE TUBES

Rescue tubes are used to help minimize personal danger when you are performing a rescue. The rescue tube is a lightweight, safe, and effective device for situations requiring rescue (**Figure 3.5**). All lifeguards must have a rescue tube at their lifeguard station.

The rescue tube provides lifeguards with several advantages when performing a rescue:

- The average rescue tube can support up to five people in the water. This greatly reduces the danger and risk to both the guest and the lifeguard during a rescue and reduces the energy you need to move the guest to safety.
- The rescue tube is positioned between the lifeguard and the guest, so the chance of the guest grabbing a lifeguard during a rescue is reduced. Even if the guest does grab a lifeguard, the rescue tube will keep them both above water.
- In the event the guest is not breathing, the rescue tube can be used to help position the guest in an open airway position if rescue breathing is started in the water.

Using the Rescue Tube While at a Lifeguard Station

How you wear or hold the rescue tube while you are on duty depends on the responsibilities of your position and the needs or regulations of the facility. A lifeguard at a wave pool must wear a rescue tube at all times, whereas a lifeguard dispatching guests at the top of a slide may not be required to wear the tube, but just have it within arm's reach where it is immediately available. The shoulder strap of the rescue tube should fit diagonally across your chest when you are wearing the tube. The following are examples

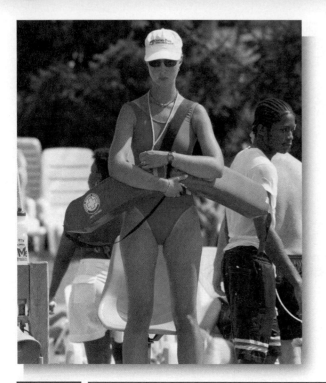

FIG 3.6   Hold the rescue tube in a manner that allows you to respond quickly to an emergency.

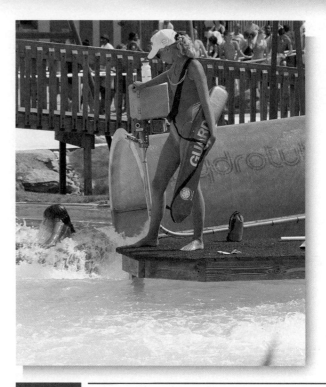

FIG 3.7   You may hold the tube at your side while standing.

of how to wear the rescue tube properly when you are on duty:

- In front of you (**Figure 3.6**)
- At your side while standing (**Figure 3.7**)
- Across your lap while sitting (**Figure 3.8**)

In all of these positions, you must secure the line (take up any slack) so that it does not get caught on anything when you move around or enter the water in an emergency.

LIFEGUARD ROTATIONS

A lifeguard **rotation** occurs when one lifeguard relieves another lifeguard at a station. The relieved lifeguard either moves to another location or goes on a break. During a rotation it is very important that proper scanning be maintained. It is easy to become distracted during the rotation. Remember that the guests are aware of your movements and the way you conduct yourself; you must always be ready to make a correction to guests' behavior or to help them should they need assistance.

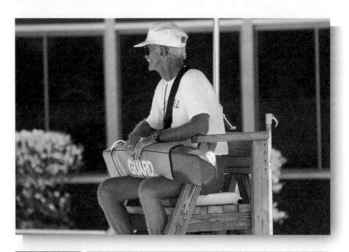

FIG 3.8   You may position the rescue tube across your lap while sitting in a chair.

During a rotation, the arriving lifeguard should walk to the next location and be on time. Conversation with the other lifeguard should be limited to pertinent information regarding the Zone of Protection area. The incoming lifeguard performs a proactive bottom scan of the zone, searching the top, middle, and bottom of the Zone of Protection area to confirm that the entire zone is clear. Make sure that the incoming lifeguard is rescue-ready

Incoming Lifeguard Has No Rescue Tube

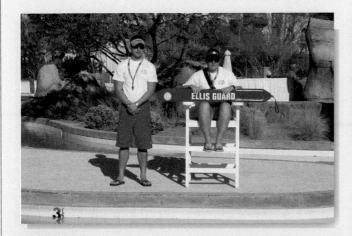

FIG 3.9a Incoming lifeguard arrives and performs a proactive bottom scan to confirm the zone is clear.

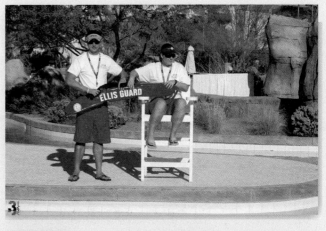

FIG 3.9b Equipment is transferred to the incoming lifeguard, and he watches the zone while the outgoing lifeguard exits the stand.

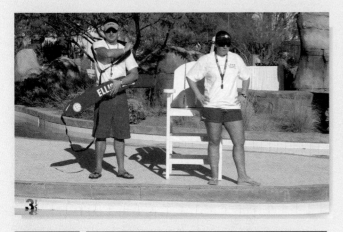

FIG 3.9c Equipment is transferred and the incoming lifeguard enters the stand while the outgoing lifeguard scans the zone.

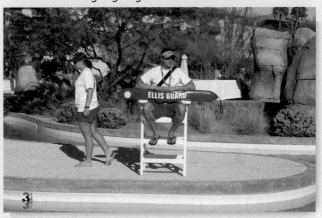

FIG 3.9d Equipment is transferred. Both lifeguards perform a proactive bottom scan before the outgoing lifeguard departs.

and has assumed responsibility for the area before the outgoing lifeguard departs. The outgoing lifeguard should also perform a complete proactive bottom scan of the zone, searching the top, middle, and bottom of the Zone of Protection area to confirm that the entire zone is clear before leaving the zone. The actions of the lifeguards during the rotation will be determined by the presence of one or two rescue tubes. For maximum protection and professionalism, conduct your rotation according to the steps identified in **Figures 3.9** and **3.10**.

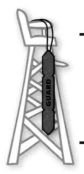

tips from the top

Stay "rescue-ready" by always having your rescue tube readily available.

Both Lifeguards Have Rescue Tubes

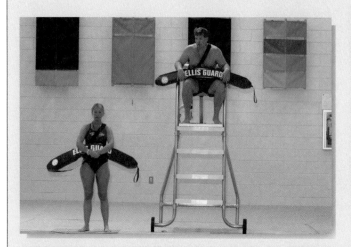

FIG 3.10a   Incoming lifeguard arrives and performs a proactive bottom scan to confirm the zone is clear.

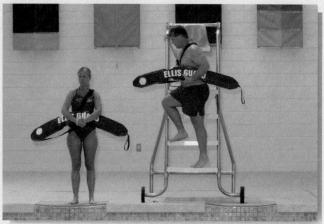

FIG 3.10b   Incoming lifeguard watches the zone while the outgoing lifeguard exits the stand.

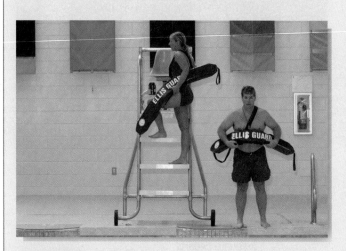

FIG 3.10c   Incoming lifeguard enters the stand while the outgoing lifeguard scans the zone.

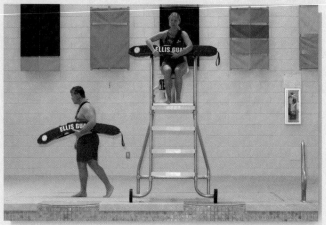

FIG 3.10d   Both lifeguards scan the zone and agree that the bottom is clear before the outgoing lifeguard departs.

~~~ WRAP-UP

Being a professional lifeguard involves:

- Working as a team to prevent drownings
- Being thoroughly familiar with your facility's emergency action plan (EAP)
- Being aware of all communication signals used at the facility
- Being prepared (rescue-ready) at all times
- Making certain all zones remain covered in the event of an emergency and during lifeguard rotations

~~~ WHAT YOU SHOULD HAVE LEARNED

After reading this chapter and completing the related course work, you should be able to:

1. Explain the purpose of an emergency action plan (EAP).
2. Identify proper precautions for assessing scene safety and Body Substance Isolation (BSI).
3. Demonstrate methods of lifeguard communication.
4. Describe the concept of team lifeguarding.
5. Identify the differences between an assist and a rescue.
6. Discuss the importance of the rescue tube.
7. Demonstrate the proper procedure for conducting a lifeguard rotation.

CHAPTER 3 Lifeguard Skills

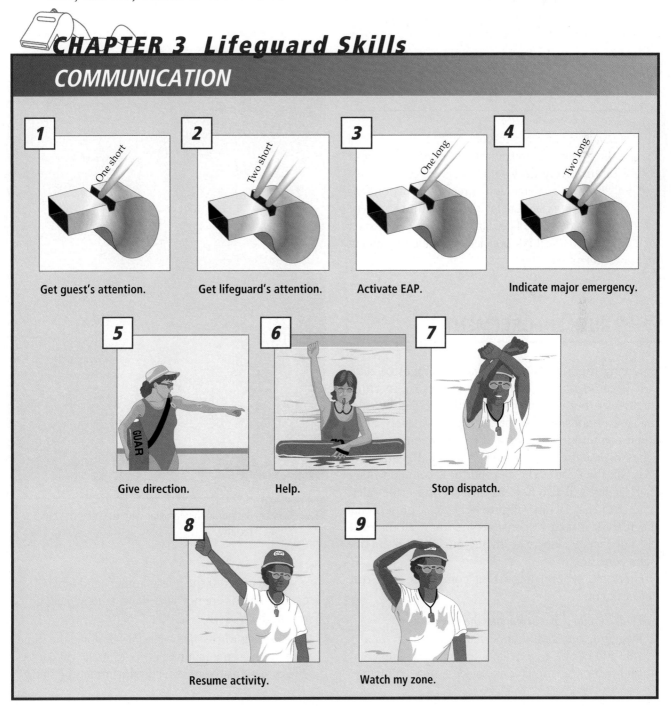

COMMUNICATION

1 One short — Get guest's attention.

2 Two short — Get lifeguard's attention.

3 One long — Activate EAP.

4 Two long — Indicate major emergency.

5 Give direction.

6 Help.

7 Stop dispatch.

8 Resume activity.

9 Watch my zone.

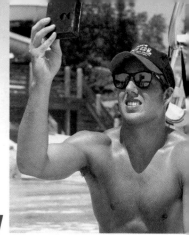

Rule Enforcement, Guest Relations, and Additional Responsibilities

〰 INTRODUCTION

As a lifeguard, your main responsibility is the safety of the guests. Part of this responsibility depends on your ability to effectively deal with guests in your facility. You will have to manage and direct their actions, as well as provide protection for their health and safety. This requires you to be familiar with the rules of your facility and your facility's policies on rule enforcement and guest relations.

〰 RULE ENFORCEMENT

Enforcing rules as a lifeguard can sometimes be difficult because people come to your facility to enjoy themselves, but your guests are still governed by rules that are established for their health and safety in an aquatic environment. Some rules are common to all types of aquatic facilities, such as "Walk" and "No Glass on the Pool Deck." Beyond these common rules, each facility will also have its own set of specific rules, unique to that facility (**Figure 4.1**). As a professional lifeguard, it is your responsibility to know all the rules of your facility, adhere to them yourself, and enforce them consistently.

There are several important components of rule enforcement:

• *Understanding and explaining the rules*—As a lifeguard, you should understand the reason for a rule and be able to explain it to guests. You may find that once you have explained a rule, enforcing

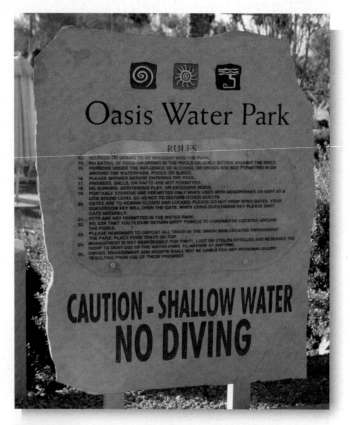

FIG 4.1 Be thoroughly familiar with the rules at your facility.

it will be easier. If the guests understand why certain actions are not safe, they are less likely to repeat them.

• *Be consistent when enforcing rules*—Enforce the same rule, in the same manner, every time. If you correct guests' actions today, you should correct the same action in the same manner tomorrow. Remember, the rules apply equally to all guests.

- *Use a positive approach*—When you make corrections, use a positive approach whenever possible. For example, instead of saying: "Don't run" say, "Please walk."

- *Be polite and respectful*—Guests respond better to positive and polite requests.

- *Know where the rules are posted*—The posted rules are a backup authority for you. Know where they are posted and refer guests to them when necessary. In larger facilities, rules are posted in several locations. There may also be specific rules for different attractions.

- *Refer problems to your supervisor*—If children keep violating a rule, have them sit for a few minutes. Sometimes a "time-out" will solve the problem. If the problem persists, or if an older guest questions or is upset about a rule, seek assistance from your supervisor. Whether that supervisor is a head lifeguard, assistant manager, or manager, it is part of his or her job to help you with rule enforcement.

〜〜 GUEST RELATIONS

Part of your responsibility as a lifeguard involves effectively dealing with guests while making them feel welcome at your facility. You will have to manage and direct their actions, as well as provide protection for their health and safety. Base your actions on the **Golden Rule of guest relations**: "Treat guests as you would like to be treated—with respect." The guests who visit your facility may be from diverse cultures and backgrounds, so you must be sensitive to their beliefs and customs. Be open to the ideas and input of guests and coworkers from various cultures. Avoid

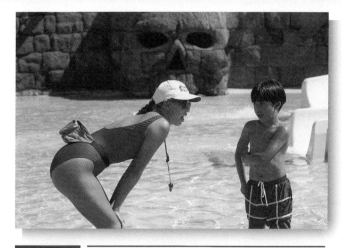

FIG 4.2 Good guest relations skills make it easier to enforce rules and create a safe and enjoyable experience for your guests.

being biased or judging others by your own background. The better your **guest relations** skills, the easier it will be for you to enforce rules and create a safe and enjoyable experience for your guests (**Figure 4.2**).

How to C.A.R.E. for Your Guests

Follow the C.A.R.E. philosophy for guest relations:

- *Confidence*—Maintain an adequate level of personal lifeguarding knowledge and skills, enhanced through appropriate initial and in-service training at your specific facility. Over time, your confidence will increase as you receive positive feedback from supervisor observations, peer review, and guest comments on your performance. Displaying a professional, enthusiastic image gives others confidence in your abilities.

- *Alertness*—Remain in a constant state of readiness. This includes focusing your attention on your guests and anticipating and preventing potential problems (e.g., weak swimmers, crowded conditions, surface glare) (**Figure 4.3**).

- *Responsiveness*—React in the appropriate manner when faced with an emergency. This includes quickly assessing a situation and determining the best course of action, including the type of response and the use of appropriate equipment.

- *Empathy*—Try to understand your guests' needs, wants, and emotions by placing yourself in their

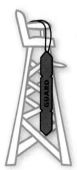

tips from the top

Remember the Golden Rule of guest relations: "Treat guests as you would like to be treated—with respect."

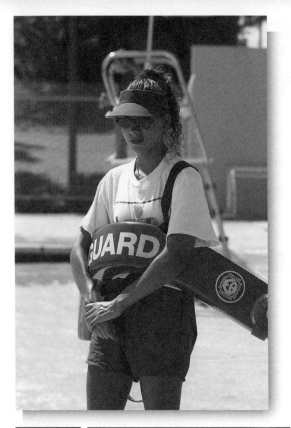

FIG 4.3 Be attentive to your guests at all times.

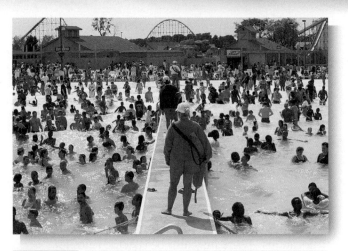

FIG 4.4   Managing large crowds during emergencies can be difficult. The EAP will guide you in emergency situations.

position. Demonstrate respect when communicating with or responding to guests and appreciate varied levels of comfort in a water environment. Understand and value any physical and emotional concerns that guests may have. Be proactive and have a positive approach to guest interactions (smile, say please and thank-you, etc.).

How to D.E.A.L. with Difficult Situations

Follow the D.E.A.L. philosophy for handling difficult situations and guests:

- *Define the problem*—Get a clear understanding of the problem. Ask questions and listen carefully to the response. Try to understand the guest's current emotional needs. Summarize the situation with those involved to be certain the problem is clearly stated. Call a supervisor for assistance, particularly if the situation will take you away from your primary lifeguard responsibilities.

- *Evaluate your options*—Examine alternatives, considering the consequences now and in the

future. Ask the guest what he or she thinks the options are to resolve the situation. When in doubt about your authority to provide options, consult a supervisor.

- *Act now*—Take action, based on the information you have acquired. Be specific when explaining to the guest what you are going to do and why you are doing it. Let everyone involved or impacted by the situation know of the action.

- *Look at outcomes*—Try to solve the problem to your and the guest's satisfaction. Sometimes the guest will not be happy with the outcome, especially if it involves a safety rule that cannot be broken. Consider ways that you could have done a better job handling this difficult guest. To avoid repeating similar circumstances, see if there is an opportunity for coworkers to learn from this situation.

Crowd Control

During an emergency, it may be necessary for you to control large numbers of guests to maintain order (**Figure 4.4**). Examples of situations where **crowd control** may be needed include severe weather conditions, chemical leaks, special events, altercations, rescues with resuscitation efforts, and terrorism threats. You should practice your emergency action plan (EAP) to be prepared for any incident requiring crowd control. Know what your responsibilities are for different events and situations, as well as where all the access and exit points are for your facility. It may sometimes be necessary to evacuate an area or open a path so that emergency medical services (EMS) personnel can reach the emergency scene.

If you need to control a crowd:

- Keep calm.
- Speak loudly and clearly.
- Give precise, simple directions.
- Speak with authority.

ADDITIONAL RESPONSIBILITIES

Paperwork

Another responsibility you will have as a lifeguard is to complete reports and maintain records. Each facility will have records and reports specific to the operation of that facility. These should include but are not limited to:

- Attendance records
- Sign-in sheets
- Maintenance schedules
- Daily work schedules
- Lifeguard rotations
- Pool chemistry records
- Weather condition reports
- In-service training records
- Incident reports

Incident reports are among the most important paperwork you will complete. Every rescue requires careful documentation. The documentation must be completed as soon as the incident has been resolved. Use the incident report forms supplied by your facility, making sure to fill in each section completely. These forms may become legal records in the future, and adequate documentation will minimize problems at that time.

Related Duties

Aquatic facilities often require lifeguards to perform duties not directly related to the primary responsibilities of preventing aquatic incidents and providing rescue and emergency care. Additional duties will vary depending on the facility and are performed during times when lifeguards are not responsible for supervising guests in the water. The duties should be provided in writing by your employer as part of your job description and/or employee orientation. These related duties may include:

- Locker room attendance
- Front desk attendance
- General facility maintenance

Maintaining Readiness

As a professional lifeguard, you should maintain your skills at "test-ready" levels at all times. The skills you learn in this course will require constant review and practice. The **in-service training** conducted at your facility will help you maintain your skill level, but it is up to you to be sure that your observation, rescue, and emergency care skills remain sharp at all times.

WRAP-UP

Being a professional lifeguard involves:

- Understanding and consistently enforcing the rules
- Being courteous to guests
- Remembering the Golden Rule of guest relations
- Processing required paperwork completely and accurately
- Maintaining readiness at all times

WHAT YOU SHOULD HAVE LEARNED

After reading this chapter and completing the related course work, you should be able to:

1. Identify ways to enforce rules.
2. Identify ways to maintain good guest relations.
3. Identify strategies for crowd control.
4. Explain the importance of paperwork and performing secondary duties.
5. Explain the importance of maintaining a high level of skill.

CHAPTER 4 Lifeguard Skills

RESPONSIBILITIES

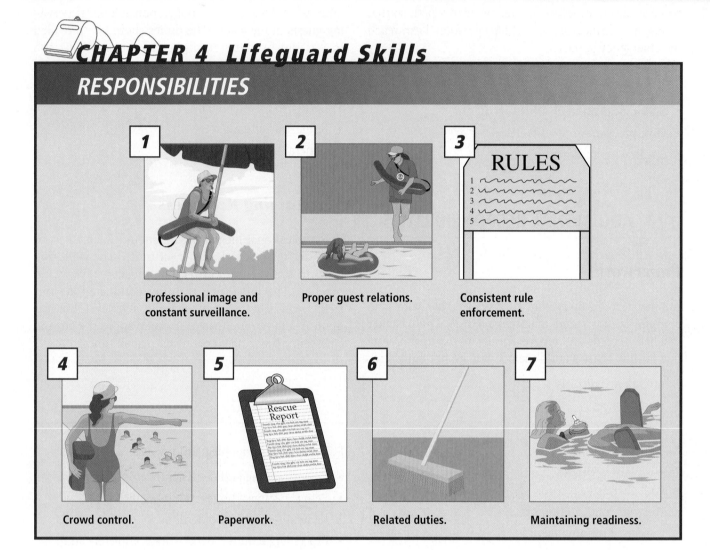

1 Professional image and constant surveillance.

2 Proper guest relations.

3 Consistent rule enforcement.

4 Crowd control.

5 Paperwork.

6 Related duties.

7 Maintaining readiness.

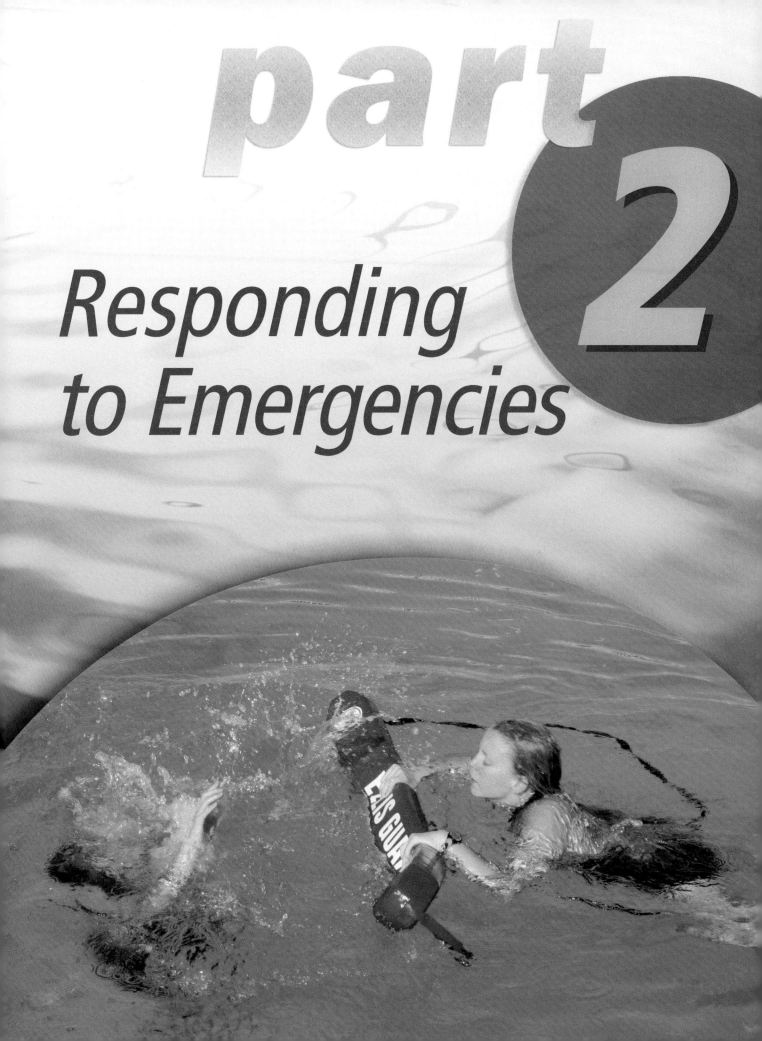

part 2

Responding to Emergencies

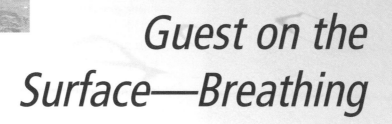

Guest on the Surface—Breathing

INTRODUCTION

This chapter introduces the skills needed to deal with water emergencies that require lifeguards to assist or rescue a guest on the surface who is still breathing.

ASSISTS

Assists involve aiding a guest, either from the deck or in the water, while still maintaining appropriate zone coverage. Guests may need an assist if they lose their footing, are slightly disoriented, have difficulty exiting the pool or standing up, or have a physical disability. You can assist these guests to safety by extending an arm or a rescue tube. It is not necessary to activate your emergency action plan (EAP) or complete a rescue report for an assist. However, if you cannot maintain proper zone coverage while assisting the guest, you must activate your EAP and execute a rescue.

Extension assists can be safely performed while standing or kneeling on the pool deck. If you are in the water (such as in a catch pool), you can also assist the guest by supporting him or her with the aid of the rescue tube. There are two common types of extensions:

- Arm extension
- Rescue tube extension

Arm Extension

To perform an arm extension:

1. Keep your body low and your center of gravity away from the water.
2. Extend your arm and grasp the guest's wrist or arm.
3. Move the guest to safety.
4. Assist the guest out of the water if appropriate.

Rescue Tube Extension

To perform a rescue tube extension (**Figure 5.1**):

1. Place the rescue tube or strap loop in the guest's hands.
2. Once the guest has a firm grasp on the tube or strap loop, move the guest to safety.
3. Assist the guest out of the water if appropriate.

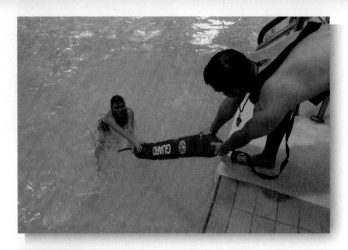

Executing a rescue tube extension.

~~~ RESCUES

A rescue occurs when you must leave your position to assist a guest and cannot maintain the proper zone coverage. Before entering the water to perform the rescue, you must activate your EAP by blowing your whistle and using the proper signal, such as pointing to the guest you will be rescuing. A rescue report must also be completed after the rescue has been accomplished. For documentation and reporting purposes, rescues are classified in one of two ways, depending on the severity of the incident:

• Distressed swimmer rescue
• Submersion incident rescue

A **distressed swimmer rescue** involves a guest who exhibits behavior indicating the inability to remain at the surface of the water or to return to the surface after submerging. The situation may result in death by drowning if the swimmer is not aided by a lifeguard.

A **submersion incident rescue** involves a guest who is rendered unconscious, submerges under water, and is rescued by a lifeguard. The situation will result in death by drowning if the swimmer is not aided by a lifeguard.

~~~ ENTRY AND APPROACH

Once you recognize that a guest is in distress:

1. Activate your EAP by blowing your whistle and pointing in the direction of the guest you are

going to rescue. This alerts other lifeguards to the area where you will be during the rescue and the need to cover your zone.

2. Push the Emergency Stop (E-Stop) button if there is one at your lifeguard station. In a wave pool, this stops the next wave from being generated. This may also notify a base station that a rescue is in progress and assistance is needed.

3. Execute a safe water entry and approach.

When entering the water and approaching a guest in distress:

• Enter the water safely using a compact jump (**Figure 5.2**).
• Maintain control of the rescue tube at all times.
• Approach the guest in a safe manner that will allow you to evaluate and control the situation.

Compact Jump Entry

When performing the **compact jump** entry:

1. Keep your eyes on the guest while preparing to jump.
2. Secure the excess line on your rescue tube so that it will not hook onto something when you jump.
3. Position the rescue tube across your chest and under your armpits.
4. Jump from the lifeguard chair or pool deck with your legs together, knees bent, and feet flat.

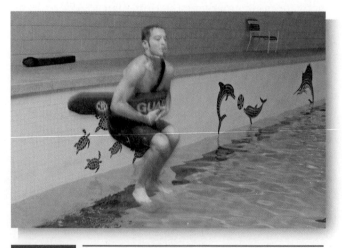

Use the compact jump when entering the water to perform a rescue.

5. You may go underneath the water briefly. The buoyancy of the rescue tube will bring you back to the surface quickly.

Approach Stroke

After entering the water, you must reach the distressed guest as quickly as possible using whatever **approach stroke** works best for you. Some lifeguards prefer to use the breaststroke (**Figure 5.3**) when approaching a guest, whereas others prefer to use the front crawl stroke (**Figure 5.4**). Use whatever combination of arm and leg movements allow you to reach the guest in the quickest and most efficient manner. As you approach, keep your eyes on the guest and the rescue tube in front of your chest; this puts you in the safest position to execute the rescue.

In some open water situations it may be faster if you allow the rescue tube to trail behind you as you swim. An example of this would be if you had to swim through a current or when entering the water from a beach and swimming a farther distance than is required or necessary in most pools. Once you get close to the distressed guest, stop, pull the rescue tube in front of you, and finish your approach.

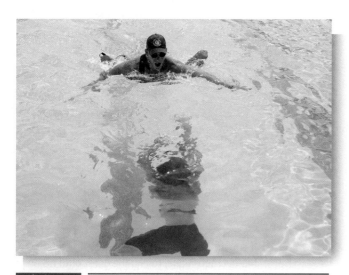

FIG 5.3 Using the breaststroke to approach a guest.

≋ EXECUTING THE RESCUE

Use one of these three methods to rescue a guest on the surface:

- Front drive rescue
- Rear hug rescue
- Two-lifeguard rescue

Front Drive Rescue

Use the **front drive rescue** when a guest is facing towards you. To execute the front drive:

1. Whistle, point to the guest, hit the E-Stop (if there is one), perform a compact jump entry, and approach stroke toward the distressed guest.

2. When you are about one body length from the guest, pull the rescue tube from under your arms and push it out in front of you with both hands (**Figure 5.5a**).

3. As you near the guest, push the tube slightly under water and drive it into the chest of the guest (**Figure 5.5b**). Keep your arms straight with your elbows locked.

4. Encourage the guest to hold on to the tube.

5. Communicate with the guest and keep kicking to maintain your momentum, moving the guest toward safety (**Figure 5.5c**).

6. Assist the guest from the water and make sure that he or she is all right before you transfer care to a supervisor and resume lifeguarding. Your EAP should explain exactly what procedure you should follow at this time, including the need to fill out a rescue report.

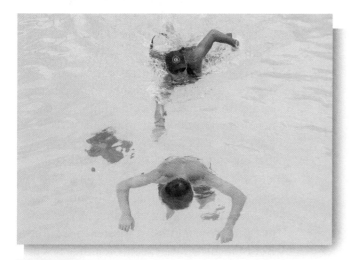

FIG 5.4 Using the front crawl stroke to approach a guest.

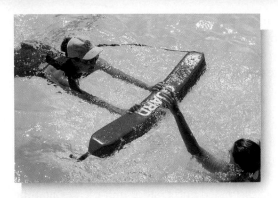

FIG 5.5a Push the rescue tube out in front of you toward the guest.

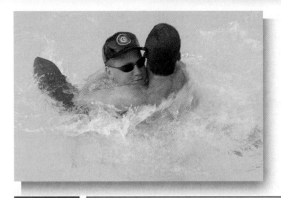

FIG 5.6 If you are grasped by the guest, use the front hug position.

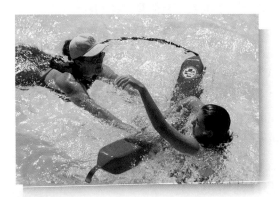

FIG 5.5b Drive the rescue tube into the guest's chest.

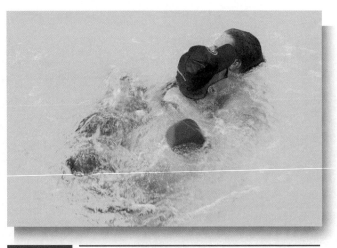

FIG 5.7 If you are being forced under water, execute the flip-over technique, rolling the guest onto his or her back.

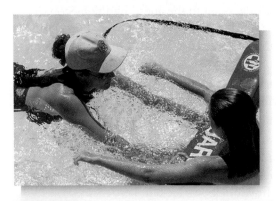

FIG 5.5c Kick to move the guest to safety.

7. If the guest should grab you during a front drive rescue, there are three modifications that may help prevent injury while still allowing you to execute an effective rescue:

- *Use a front hug position.* Keep the rescue tube between you and the guest. If your head is still above water after the guest grabs you, continue to move toward an exit or the side

of the pool. Reach under the guest's arms and hug the guest. Keep your head slightly to the side of the guest so he or she cannot hurt you if his or her head moves quickly toward you (**Figure 5.6**).

- *Use a flip-over technique.* Keep the rescue tube between you and the guest. If you are being forced underwater, execute a flip-over to position yourself on top of the guest. This puts the guest on his or her back. Keep kicking and moving forward (**Figure 5.7**).

- *Use a push-away.* If you cannot control the situation because of the way the guest has grabbed you, you are choking, or you have lost your rescue tube, it is safer to separate from the guest and execute another rescue. To execute a push-away, get some air, tuck your chin, and submerge. Push yourself away from the guest, recover your rescue

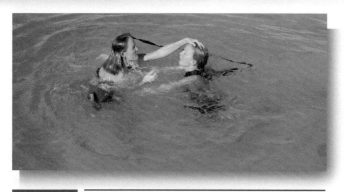

FIG 5.8a Push-away technique.

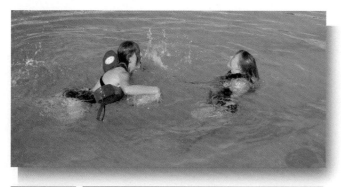

FIG 5.8b Tuck your chin, submerge, and push-away from the guest.

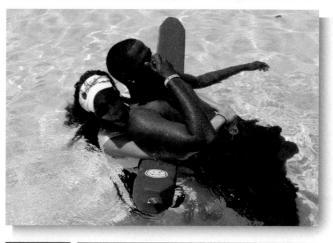

FIG 5.9a Perform the rear hug.

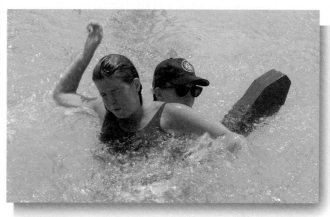

FIG 5.9b Keep your body and head to the side in case the guest panics.

tube, position it between you and the guest, and re-approach the guest or signal for help from a second lifeguard (**Figure 5.8**).

Rear Hug

Use the **rear hug rescue** when a guest is facing away from you. To execute the rear hug:

1. Whistle, point to the guest, hit the E-Stop (if there is one), perform a compact jump entry, and approach stroke to a position directly behind the distressed guest, keeping the rescue tube against your chest and under your arms.

2. Bring your body to a neutral (vertical) position in the water before initiating contact with the distressed guest. Extend your arms under the guest's armpits and wrap your hands around his or her chest to elevate the guest above the surface of the water (**Figure 5.9a**). Alternatively, you may place your arms around the guest's waist to enable you to lift him or her higher above the surface.

3. Keep your body and head slightly to the side of the guest. Either lean in close or lean

back comfortably to avoid injury should the guest snap his or her head back suddenly (**Figure 5.9b**).

4. Communicate with the guest and keep kicking to maintain your momentum, moving the guest to safety.

5. Assist the guest from the water and make sure that he or she is all right before you transfer care to a supervisor and resume lifeguarding. Your EAP should explain exactly what procedure you should follow at this time, including the need to fill out a rescue report.

Two-Lifeguard Rescue

Use the **two-lifeguard rescue** when a distressed guest is too active for one lifeguard to handle safely. The two-lifeguard rescue involves simultaneously placing two rescue tubes against the guest, one against the chest and the other against the back. To execute the two-lifeguard rescue:

1. The primary rescuer raises a fist above his or her head to indicate the need for assistance from a back-up lifeguard (**Figure 5.10a**).

2. The back-up lifeguard blows his or her whistle. Both lifeguards perform compact jump entries and approach the guest from opposite sides.

3. Communication between the lifeguards is very important as they prepare to make contact with the guest.

4. At the signal to move, the lifeguard behind the distressed guest executes a rear hug, and the lifeguard in front of the guest executes a front drive (**Figure 5.10b**). The lifeguard executing the rear hug presents a target for the lifeguard in front of the guest to place the rescue tube against.

5. As the front lifeguard executes the front drive, the rear lifeguard reaches over the rescue tube and pulls it against the chest of the guest. This "sandwiches" the guest between the two rescue tubes and lifeguards (**Figure 5.10c**).

6. Both lifeguards move the guest to safety while providing reassurance.

7. Assist the guest from the water and make sure that he or she is all right before you transfer care to a supervisor and resume lifeguarding. Your EAP should explain exactly what procedure you should follow at this time, including the need to fill out a rescue report.

Dealing with Multiple Guests in Distress

From time to time, lifeguards may encounter multiple swimmers who need assistance at the same time. These instances typically occur in attractions with moving water or current or in open water environments; when one guest in distress grabs on to another swimmer; or when one swimmer attempts to help another and both end up in distress. As a lifeguard you should be prepared to handle rescue situations involving more than one guest in distress. To execute rescues of multiple guests in distress, you must keep the big picture objectives in mind: maintain your own safety and provide assistance to all guests in distress by enabling

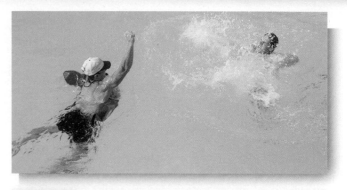

FIG 5.10a Signal for assistance from a second lifeguard.

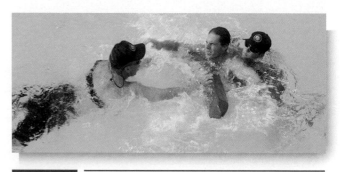

FIG 5.10b In the two-lifeguard rescue, the rear lifeguard executes a rear hug, while the front lifeguard executes a front drive.

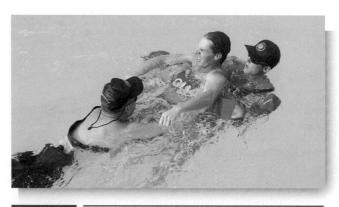

FIG 5.10c The guest is "sandwiched" between the two rescue tubes and lifeguards and moved to safety.

them to remain at the surface. Multiple guests in distress rescues are situations where the "make it work" philosophy is often necessary. To execute a rescue for multiple guests in distress:

1. The primary lifeguard activates the EAP and signals for assistance by raising a fist above his or her head.

2. The back-up lifeguard accounts for the safety of the remaining swimmers and/or clears the Zone of Protection area.

3. The primary lifeguard performs an appropriate rescue of the first guest in distress encountered.

4. Once the first guest in distress is secured on the rescue tube, the lifeguard proceeds to the next guest in distress and renders aid by whatever means is practical, using the rescue tube as much as possible.

5. When the zone is clear or additional staff has responded to take over zone responsibilities, a secondary lifeguard enters the water and provides assistance to the primary lifeguard.

6. The lifeguards should move the guests to safety while providing reassurance.

7. The lifeguards assist the guests from the water and make sure that they are all right

before transferring care to a supervisor and resuming lifeguard duties. The EAP should explain exactly what procedures to follow at this time, including the need to fill out a rescue report.

≈≈≈ WRAP-UP

Being a professional lifeguard involves:

- Understanding when to use an assist and when to use a rescue
- Entering the water in a safe manner at all times
- Communicating with other lifeguards
- Performing the appropriate rescue for the situation, in a manner that is both safe and effective

≈≈≈ WHAT YOU SHOULD HAVE LEARNED

After reading this chapter and completing the related course work, you should be able to:

1. Demonstrate a compact jump entry.
2. Demonstrate a safe and controlled approach.
3. Perform a front drive, rear hug, and two-lifeguard rescue.
4. Perform a rescue of multiple guests in distress.

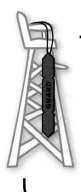

tips from the top

Do not be afraid to request assistance when needed. Practice the two-lifeguard rescue to get your timing down. You should also practice rescuing multiple guests in distress at the same time.

CHAPTER 5 Lifeguard Skills

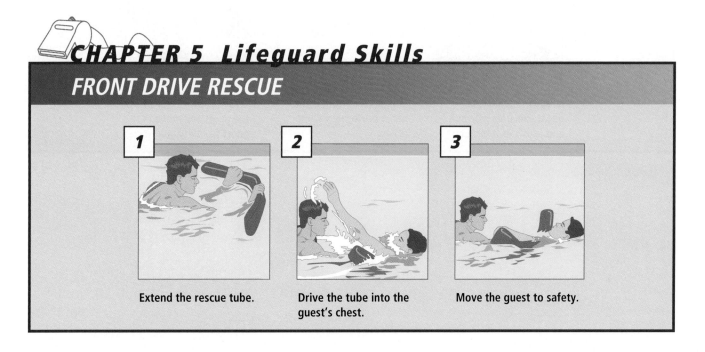

FRONT DRIVE RESCUE

1 Extend the rescue tube.

2 Drive the tube into the guest's chest.

3 Move the guest to safety.

CHAPTER 5 Lifeguard Skills

REAR HUG RESCUE

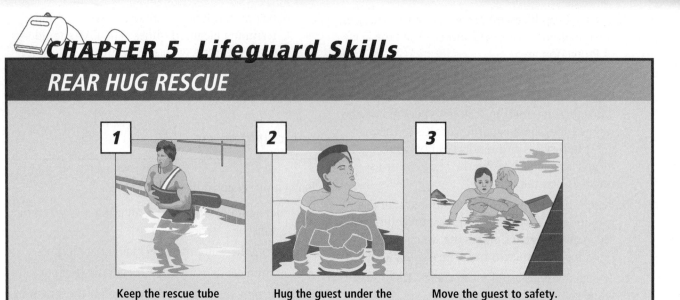

1 Keep the rescue tube against your chest and under your arms.

2 Hug the guest under the armpits.

3 Move the guest to safety.

CHAPTER 5 Lifeguard Skills

TWO-LIFEGUARD RESCUE

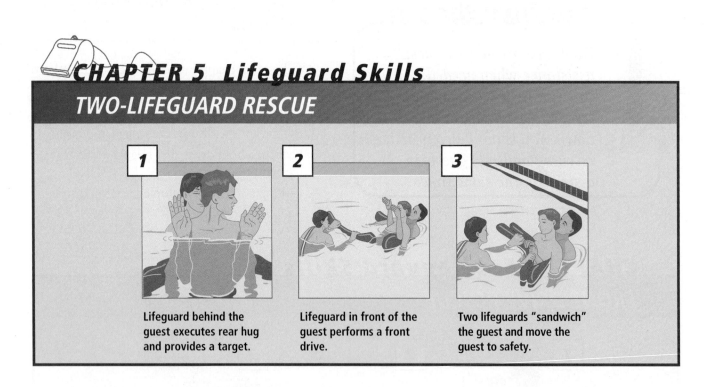

1 Lifeguard behind the guest executes rear hug and provides a target.

2 Lifeguard in front of the guest performs a front drive.

3 Two lifeguards "sandwich" the guest and move the guest to safety.

Rescue Breathing and Airway Management

≈≈ INTRODUCTION

The successful resuscitation of a submerged guest who is not breathing begins with an understanding of basic airway and ventilation management skills. These life-saving skills are presented in this chapter and should be reviewed regularly during periodic in-service training sessions.

≈≈ RESPONSIVENESS AND BREATHING

If a guest is conscious and talking, then the guest is said to be responsive. Ask the guest his or her name and what happened. If the guest responds appropriately, then he or she is alert.

If the guest lies motionless and does not respond, tap the guest's shoulder and ask, "Are you okay?" If there is no response, the guest is considered unresponsive (unconscious). If the guest is unresponsive, assess his or her breathing and activate the EAP (**Figure 6.1**).

If the guest is breathing normally place him or her in the recovery position and provide care based upon the signs and symptoms found. If the guest is not breathing, breathing abnormally (e.g. gasping), or the rescuer is uncertain if the guest is breathing adequately, the rescuer should proceed to check for a pulse.

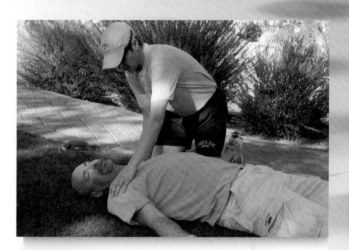

FIG 6.1 Determine responsiveness and check breathing.

≈≈ PULSE

Check for a pulse in the carotid artery in the neck (adult or child) or brachial artery in the arm (infant) for up to 10 seconds. If the pulse is absent, barely detectable, or if the rescuer is uncertain, begin CPR. CPR is covered in Chapter 7.

If a pulse is present, but the guest is not breathing, open the guest's airway and begin rescue breathing.

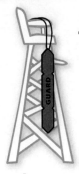

tips from the top

When checking breathing, keep in mind that an unresponsive (unconscious) guest may have occasional gasping breaths called <u>agonal breaths</u>, which occur in the first few minutes of cardiac arrest. These are ineffective ventilations and should not be confused with adequate breathing. In these cases, rescue breathing should be provided to the guest (or perform CPR, if pulse is absent).

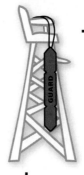

tips from the top

Guests injured in diving incidents, showing signs of head or neck injury, or complaining of head, neck, or back pain must be cared for as if a possible spinal cord injury has occurred. In this case, the head and neck should be stabilized and the airway opened using the jaw-thrust without head tilt technique.

Jaw-Thrust with Head Tilt

To perform the <u>jaw-thrust with head tilt</u> technique (**Figure 6.2**):

1. Kneel at the top of the guest's head.
2. Hook your index and middle fingers of each hand behind the angle of the guest's jaw, and place your thumbs on the guest's cheekbones.
3. Lift the jaw with your fingers while pressing down with your thumbs.
4. Tilt the head back.

Jaw-Thrust Without Head Tilt

To perform the <u>jaw-thrust without head tilt</u> technique (**Figure 6.3**):

1. Kneel at the top of the guest's head.
2. Hook your index and middle fingers of each hand behind the angle of the guest's jaw, and place your thumbs on the guest's cheekbones.
3. Lift the jaw with your fingers while pressing down with your thumbs. Do not tilt the head back.

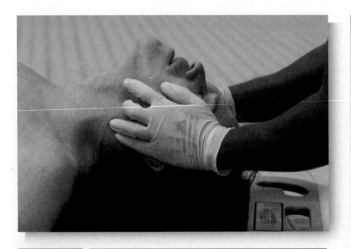

FIG 6.2 Jaw-thrust with head tilt.

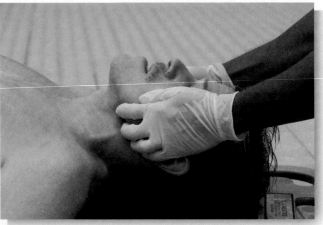

FIG 6.3 Jaw-thrust without head tilt.

Recovery Position

The <u>recovery position</u> can be used to assist an unconscious guest who is breathing or vomiting if you do not suspect spinal injury. The recovery position uses gravity to help move the guest's tongue away from the back of the throat and allows for the passive drainage of fluids from the mouth (**Figure 6.4**). Log roll the body as a unit, moving the head, shoulders, and hips together.

≈≈ RESCUE BREATHING

If the guest is not breathing, you should begin the process of <u>rescue breathing</u>. Rescue breathing requires you to give breaths to the guest so that the guest's chest gently rises. Although rescue breathing can be done through mouth-to-mouth contact, lifeguards should provide rescue breathing only through a barrier device such as a resuscitation mask to lower the risk of exposure to infectious diseases.

Each rescue breath (ventilation) should take 1 second. When initiating rescue breathing, give 2 initial ventilations. Give 1 normal breath approximately every 5 seconds. For children or infants, give 1 normal breath every 3 seconds. Do this for approximately 2 minutes, then recheck the guest's <u>pulse</u>.

Using a Resuscitation Mask

A <u>resuscitation mask</u> allows you to ventilate a nonbreathing guest by covering his or her mouth and nose with a clear plastic mask and breathing through a one-way valve (**Figure 6.5**). There are many types of

resuscitation masks, face shields, and bag valve masks (see Chapter 8). Some have separate one-way valves, while others have the valves attached. The mask and valve eliminate direct mouth-to-mouth contact between you and the guest and can divert the guest's exhaled air away from you.

Clear masks are required so that the lifeguard can see any vomit or other obstructions in the guest's airway. It is also recommended to use a mask that can be connected to a supplemental oxygen source in case the guest needs additional oxygen during the process of rescue breathing (**Figure 6.6**). Finally, the mask should

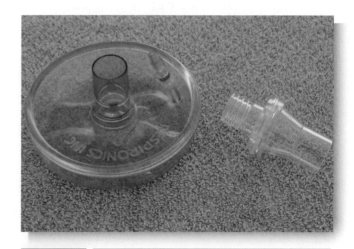

FIG 6.5 Resuscitation mask with one-way valve.

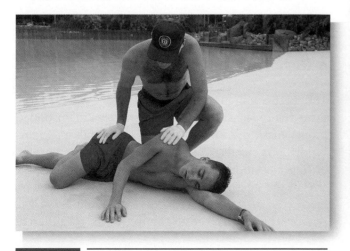

FIG 6.4 Recovery position.

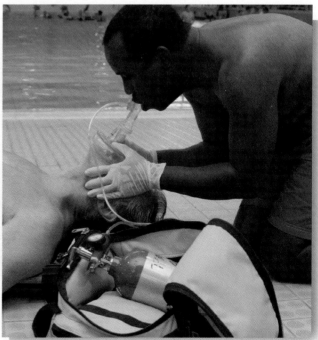

FIG 6.6 Resuscitation mask attached to oxygen.

allow a practice guest in distress to breathe while the mask is sealed on the face.

To use a resuscitation mask once you have determined that a guest is not breathing, but has a definite pulse:

1. Examine the mask to make sure that it is adequately inflated to provide a good seal over the guest's face.

2. Attach the one-way valve to the mask (if not already attached).

3. Place the mask on the guest's face so that it covers the nose and mouth (**Figure 6.7**). Place your thumbs on the mask, over the guest's cheekbones. Place your index fingers behind the angles of the guest's jaw.

4. Perform the jaw-thrust technique with or without head tilt, depending on the guest's condition.

5. Seal the mask to the guest's face.

6. Take a normal breath and breathe into the one-way valve. Each rescue breath should last approximately 1 second. You should see the chest rise with each breath you provide (**Figure 6.8**).

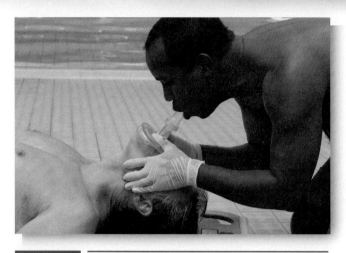

FIG 6.8   Providing rescue breaths through a resuscitation mask.

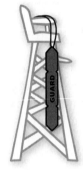

tips from the top

*Another option when using a resuscitation mask is to kneel at the side of the guest's head and apply the mask over the guest's face. Use both hands to maintain a seal on the mask and tilt the guest's head back. This position works well if you are a lone rescuer and the guest also needs CPR; it is **not** recommended in team management situations.*

Complications of Using a Resuscitation Mask

The most common problem rescuers face when using a resuscitation mask is the inability to maintain both a proper mask seal and an open airway while providing ventilations/breaths. You may need to adjust your hand or finger position based on the size of your hands, the size of the guest's head, and the type of resuscitation mask you are using. As part of your training you will practice placing the resuscitation mask on different

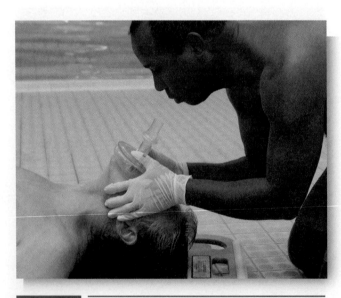

FIG 6.7   Applying a resuscitation mask for rescue breathing.

people and manikins on land and in the water. This will help you master this skill in a variety of situations.

~~~ FOREIGN BODY AIRWAY OBSTRUCTION (FBAO)

A guest's airway may be obstructed by a **foreign body** (like a small piece of food). The foreign matter must be removed before rescue breathing will be effective.

Recognizing Foreign Body Airway Obstruction (Choking)

A foreign body lodged in the airway may cause a mild or severe airway obstruction. In a mild (partial) airway obstruction, good air exchange is present, so the guest is able to make forceful coughing efforts in an attempt to relieve the obstruction. The guest should be encouraged to cough, because this is likely to remove the obstruction.

A guest with a severe airway obstruction will have poor air exchange. Signs of severe (complete) airway obstruction include:

- Difficult or strained breathing
- Weak, ineffective cough
- Inability to speak
- Bluish-gray coloring on skin, fingernail beds, or inside of mouth
- Hands clutched at throat, demonstrating the universal chocking sign of distress (**Figure 6.9**)

Caring for an Airway Obstruction in a Responsive Adult or Child

To determine if care is needed, ask the guest, "Are you choking?" If the guest is able to verbally respond, encourage the guest to cough to remove the mild (partial) obstruction. If the guest is unable to respond verbally, but nods "yes," then provide care for a severe airway obstruction by performing the **Heimlich maneuver**.

To perform the Heimlich maneuver:

1. Place your fist against the guest's abdomen, with your thumb just above the guest's navel.

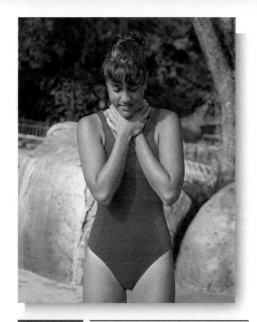

FIG 6.9   The universal choking sign.

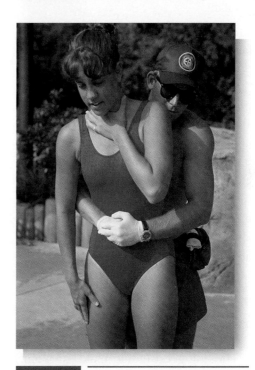

FIG 6.10   Perform the Heimlich maneuver for responsive choking adults or children.

2. Grasp the fist with your other hand and press into the guest's abdomen using quick inward and upward thrusts (**Figure 6.10**).

3. Continue **abdominal thrusts** until the object is removed or the guest becomes unconscious.

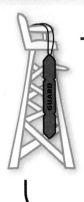

tips from the top

To clear an airway obstruction in a responsive guest who is pregnant or obese, place your hands on the center of the chest (instead of the abdomen) and give chest thrusts to remove the foreign object.

Sometimes a ventilation may not enter the lungs of an unresponsive guest. In this case, reposition the airway and try an additional ventilation. In most cases, this will resolve the issue. If the second ventilation still does not enter the lungs, assume the airway is obstructed and begin 30 chest compressions followed by 2 ventilations. Each time the airway is opened prior to giving ventilations, look for an object in the mouth. If an object is visible, remove it with a finger sweep and then attempt the ventilations. Once the ventilations go in, resume care of the guest.

Caring for an Airway Obstruction in a Responsive Infant

The Heimlich maneuver should not be used for infants under one year old. To remove an airway obstruction in a responsive infant:

1. Supporting the infant's head and neck, lay the infant face down on your forearm and lower your arm to your leg.
2. Firmly administer five back blows between the infant's shoulder blades with the heel of your hand (**Figure 6.11**).
3. Holding the infant securely with your forearms, support the back of the infant's head and roll the infant face up.
4. Firmly give five chest thrusts on the infant's sternum, between the nipple line (**Figure 6.12**).
5. Repeat these steps until the object is removed or the infant becomes unresponsive (unconscious).

Caring for an Airway Obstruction in an Unresponsive Guest

If a responsive choking guest (adult, child, or infant) becomes unresponsive, the guest should be lowered to the ground and chest compressions should be started immediately (see Chapter 7). After performing 30 chest compressions, open the airway and check for a foreign object before giving 2 ventilations.

If an object is visible, remove it with a finger sweep, simply by inserting your gloved finger into the mouth and scooping out the object. The finger sweep should not be used with infants; instead, the object should be plucked out.

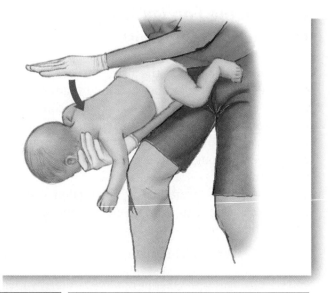

FIG 6.11 Back blows for a responsive choking infant.

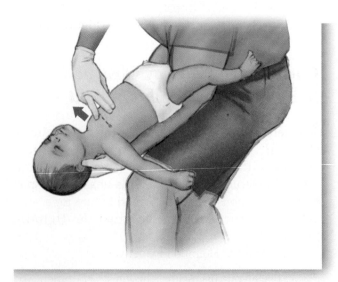

FIG 6.12 Chest thrusts for a responsive choking infant.

Using a Manual Suction Device

If an unresponsive (unconscious) guest begins to vomit, you will need to keep the guest's airway clear. Roll the guest into the recovery position to allow fluid/vomit to flow out of the mouth (**Figure 6.13**). Take extra precautions to keep the head and neck of guests with suspected head/neck injury in alignment. You can insert a gloved finger and attempt to sweep solid objects from the mouth as needed. When available, a manual (hand-operated) suction device should be used to remove the fluid/vomit from the guest's mouth during resuscitation (**Figure 6.14**).

To use a manual suction device:

1. Roll the guest to one side and perform a finger sweep until a suction device is available.
2. Install a new cartridge into the suction device if necessary.
3. Remove the protective cap from the tip of the suction catheter.
4. Open the guest's mouth and insert the catheter to the base of the tongue.
5. Squeeze the suction handle and hold until suction stops. Repeat as needed.
6. Suction no longer than 10 seconds.
7. Once you have completed care for the guest, dispose of the cartridge as biohazard waste.

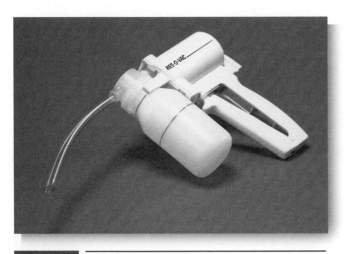

FIG 6.13 Roll the guest to one side and perform a finger sweep until a suction device is available.

～～WRAP-UP

Being a professional lifeguard involves:

- Determining responsiveness and normal breathing
- Understanding when and how to open a blocked airway
- Being able to provide effective rescue breathing using a resuscitation mask
- Being able to remove foreign body airway obstructions

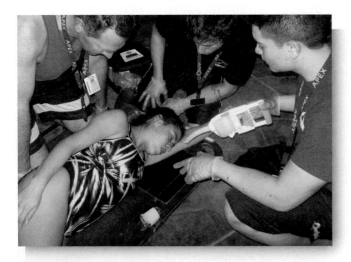

FIG 6.14 Handheld suction device.

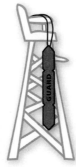

tips from the top

Leave the stroke adjustment of the suction device in position for maximum pressure. The handheld suction device is not intended for use with infants or young children. Let the size of the guest's mouth be a guide as to when to use the device. Never force the catheter into the mouth.

～～ WHAT YOU SHOULD HAVE LEARNED

After reading this chapter and completing the related course work, you should be able to:

1. Demonstrate how to open a guest's airway using the jaw-thrust (with or without head tilt).
2. Demonstrate how to place a guest in the recovery position.
3. Perform rescue breathing using a resuscitation mask.
4. Remove a foreign body airway obstruction from an adult, child, or infant.
5. Use a manual suction device.

CHAPTER 6 Lifeguard Skills

RESCUE BREATHING AND AIRWAY MANAGEMENT

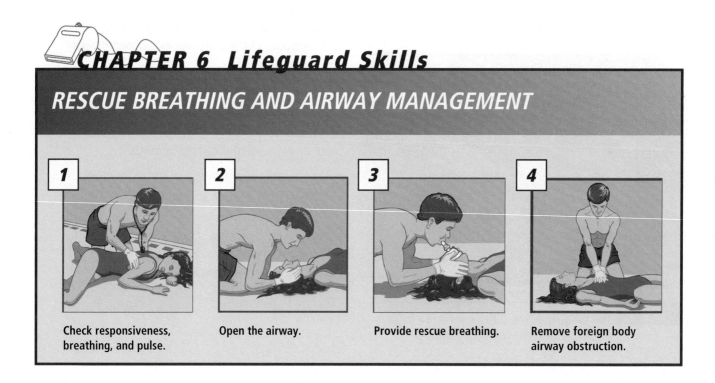

1 Check responsiveness, breathing, and pulse.

2 Open the airway.

3 Provide rescue breathing.

4 Remove foreign body airway obstruction.

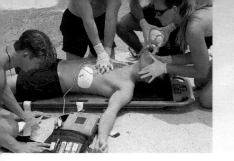

CPR and AED

INTRODUCTION: HOW THE HEART WORKS

The heart is an organ with four hollow chambers (**Figure 7.1**). The two right-side chambers receive oxygen-poor blood from the body and pump it out to the lungs, where waste products are removed and oxygen is introduced. This oxygen-rich blood is returned to the two chambers on the left side of the heart, where it is pumped out to the rest of the body.

To ensure healthy blood circulation and heart functioning, the muscles of these chambers have to work together. They are controlled by a small collection of special pacemaker cells that are found in the upper right chamber of the heart and emit electrical impulses to all the heart muscle cells. These electrical impulses keep the heart beating regularly.

CARDIAC ARREST

When the heart's electrical and mechanical system malfunctions, the heart stops beating. This condition is called <u>cardiac arrest</u>. At this point, blood stops circulating, the oxygen supply is cut off from the body, and no signs of life are visible. Without immediate treatment, cardiac arrest leads to death.

Many sudden cardiac arrest victims have an electrical malfunction of the heart called <u>ventricular fibrillation</u> (V-fib) in which the electrical impulses become chaotic and the heart's pumping function abruptly ceases (**Figure 7.2**). Another common cause of cardiac arrest is <u>ventricular tachycardia</u> (V-tach), in which the heart beats too quickly to pump blood effectively (**Figure 7.3**). Both conditions are extremely serious and demand immediate care.

Care for Cardiac Arrest

Time is a crucial factor in situations of cardiac arrest, and all components of care should be administered as soon as possible. To care for cardiac arrest, lifeguards should follow the four-step "chain of cardiac care" (**Figure 7.4**):

1. *Emergency action plan (EAP)*—Activate the EAP to indicate to other lifeguards that there is an emergency and that assistance will be needed.

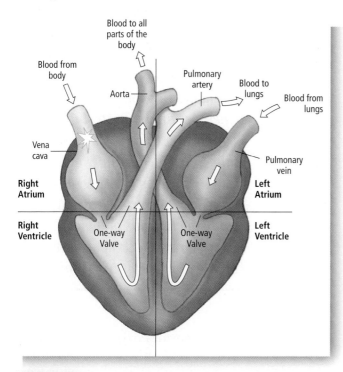

FIG 7.1   The four chambers of the human heart.

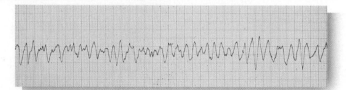

FIG 7.2 Ventricular fibrillation is chaotic electrical activity.

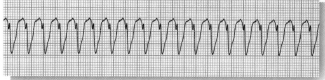

FIG 7.3 Ventricular tachycardia is very rapid electrical activity.

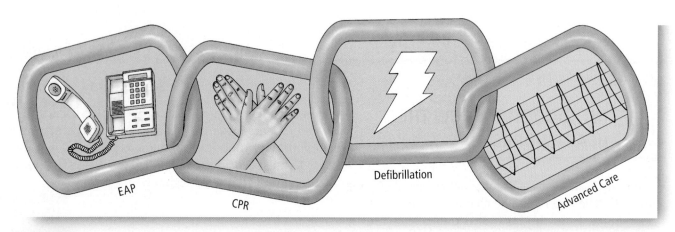

Defibrillation

EAP

CPR

Advanced Care

FIG 7.4 Links in the chain of cardiac care.

2. *CPR*—Perform <u>cardiopulmonary resuscitation (CPR)</u>, a combination of rescue breathing and chest compressions, to help temporarily supply oxygen to the brain and "buy time" until more advanced medical care can be provided.

3. *Defibrillation*—Defibrillation provides an electrical shock to the heart in order to re-establish a healthy heart rhythm resulting in normal electrical and pumping functions. This shock is delivered by an electrical device known as an <u>automated external defibrillator (AED)</u>.

4. *Advanced care*—Specially trained medical personnel will be needed to treat a guest in cardiac arrest. Even if defibrillation is successful, advanced care will be required.

CARDIOPULMONARY RESUSCITATION (CPR)

"Cardio" refers to the heart, and "pulmonary" refers to the lungs. Cardiopulmonary resuscitation (CPR) is a combination of chest compressions (which keep the heart circulating blood throughout the body) and res-

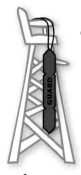

tips from the top

There are slight variations in CPR techniques for adults, children, and infants. Although CPR skills are not difficult to learn, these techniques may be difficult to remember after your training. It is important to practice these skills frequently so that you can recall them easily during an emergency. In-service training and frequent skills audits will help you remain competent and confident with your CPR skills.

cue breathing (which provides oxygen to the lungs). CPR is an important step of early care to help sustain victims of cardiac arrest until more advanced medical care can be provided (**Figure 7.5**).

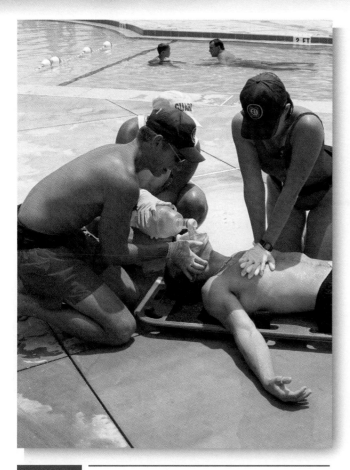

FIG 7.5 Lifeguards often perform CPR as part of a team response to an emergency.

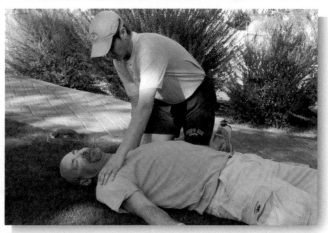

FIG 7.6 Check for responsiveness and breathing.

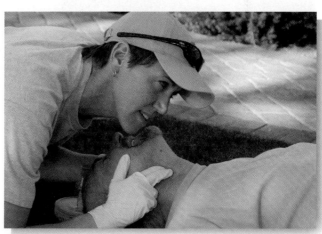

FIG 7.7 Check for a pulse.

Assessing the Situation

As always, assess the scene safety first and take proper BSI precautions before contacting the guest.

1. Check responsiveness by tapping the guest and shouting, "Are you okay?". At the same time, check quickly for breathing (**Figure 7.6**).

2. If the guest does not respond, activate the EAP to retrieve an AED.

3. If the guest is breathing and no spinal injury is suspected, roll him or her into the recovery position.

4. If the guest is not breathing or breathing is inadequate, check for a pulse (**Figure 7.7**). For adults or children, place your fingers on either side of the neck near the carotid artery. For infants, place your fingers on the inside of the upper arm near the brachial artery. Check the pulse for up to 10 seconds.

5. If there is a pulse but the guest is not breathing adequately, open the airway and provide rescue breathing (1 ventilation approximately every 5 seconds for adults and 1 ventilation every 3 seconds for children and infants) for 2 minutes, and then recheck the pulse.

6. If there is no pulse and no breathing, begin CPR.

Adult, One-Rescuer CPR

1. Place the heel of one hand on the center of the chest between the nipples. Place the other hand on top of the first.
2. Depress the chest 2 inches.
3. Give 30 chest compressions at a rate of at least 100 per minute (**Figure 7.8**).

4. Open the airway, and give 2 breaths (1 second each) (**Figure 7.9**).
5. Continue cycles of 30 chest compressions and 2 breaths until an AED is available or EMS personnel arrive and take over.
6. Apply the AED and follow its prompts.

Child, One-Rescuer CPR

1. Place the heel of one or two hands on the center of the chest between the nipples.
2. Depress the chest ⅓ of its total depth, using one hand or two hands (as necessary to achieve proper depth of 2 inches).
3. Give 30 chest compressions at a rate of at least 100 per minute (**Figure 7.10**).
4. Open the airway, and give 2 breaths (1 second each).
5. Continue cycles of 30 chest compressions and 2 breaths until an AED is available or EMS personnel arrive and take over.
6. Apply the AED and follow its prompts.

Infant, One-Rescuer CPR

1. Place 2 fingers on the breastbone just below the nipple line.
2. Depress the chest ⅓ the depth of the chest (1½ inches).

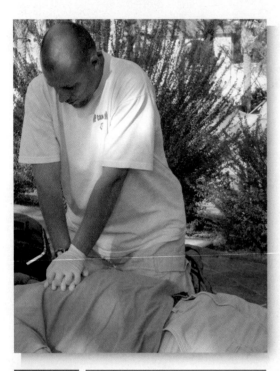

FIG 7.8   Adult CPR.

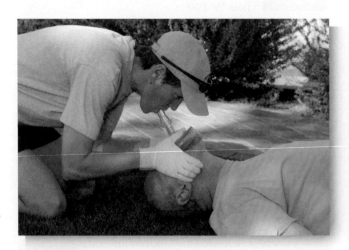

FIG 7.9   Open the airway and provide ventilations.

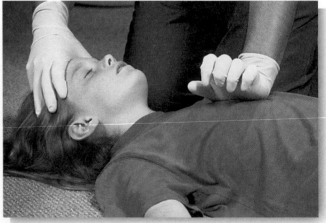

FIG 7.10   Child CPR.

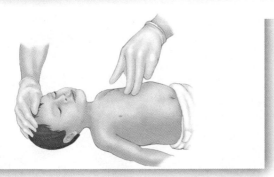

FIG 7.11 Infant CPR.

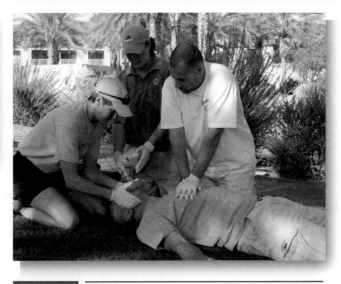

FIG 7.12 Multiple-rescuer CPR.

3. Give 30 chest compressions at a rate of at least 100 per minute (**Figure 7.11**).

4. Open the airway, and give 2 breaths (1 second each).

5. Continue cycles of 30 chest compressions and 2 breaths until an AED is available or EMS personnel arrive and take over.

6. Apply the AED and follow its prompts.

Multiple-Rescuer CPR

In most emergency situations, more than one lifeguard will be involved. The tasks of providing chest compressions and rescue breathing are physically demanding. Two or more lifeguards working as a team during CPR can help reduce fatigue and improve the efficiency and quality of compressions. Therefore, it is recommended that multiple-rescuer CPR be performed whenever possible.

When performing multiple-rescuer CPR, one lifeguard will provide chest compressions while another performs ventilations (**Figure 7.12**). After about 2 minutes of care, or once the AED prompts rescuers to stand clear for analysis, rescuers should switch positions so that compressions can be continued with a fresh lifeguard. This will ensure appropriate chest compression depth and rate. Do not hesitate to ask for relief at any time when you are performing CPR.

In multiple-rescuer CPR, the ratio of compressions to ventilations will be different for infants and children than in one-rescuer CPR. When performing multiple-rescuer CPR on infants and children, rescuers should perform cycles of 15 chest compressions (rather than 30 compressions, as in one-rescuer CPR) and 2 breaths.

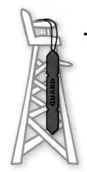

tips from the top

When performing multiple-rescuer CPR on an infant, the two-thumb technique is preferable, with the hands encircling the infant's chest. This method has been shown to provide better blood flow than the two-finger method.

DEFIBRILLATION

Although CPR can help "buy time," defibrillation is necessary to restore normal heart function following cardiac arrest. **Defibrillation** delivers an electrical shock to the heart, momentarily stopping all electrical activity. When the electrical impulses of the special pacemaker cells resume, the heart may return to normal beating and blood circulation. More than one shock may be necessary to produce this effect, and in some cases defibrillation may not be successful due to heart muscle damage or other underlying factors.

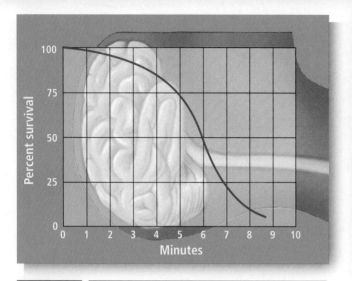

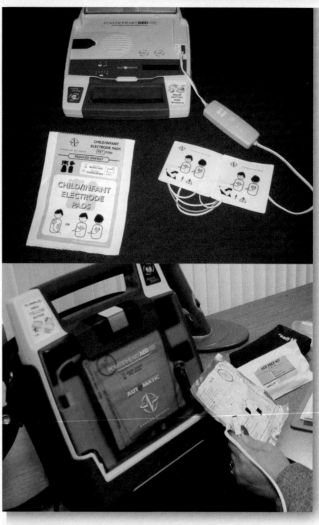

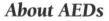
FIG 7.13 A guest's chance of survival decreases with every minute that passes without proper care.

During cardiac arrest, early care is essential to increase the chances of survival. For every minute that defibrillation is delayed, the guest's chance of survival decreases 7 to 10 percent (**Figure 7.13**). The development of the automated external defibrillator (AED) has helped make early defibrillation possible with only minimal training. An AED can analyze the heart's rhythm, determine when defibrillation is needed, and administer shock to correct electrical disturbances and end cardiac arrest. In combination with early CPR, AEDs help save thousands of lives every year.

FIG 7.14 AED devices have similar features and can be used on adults, children, and infants.

About AEDs

There are several different kinds of AEDs, but the basic principles of operation are always the same. An AED contains a cable that is connected to two adhesive pads (electrodes) (**Figure 7.14**). These pads are placed on the guest's bare, dry chest and create a circuit to send an electrical signal from the heart into the device for analysis and then deliver an electric shock to the guest if needed. AEDs also record the guest's heart rhythm, known as an electrocardiogram (ECG), shock data, and other information about device performance (e.g., date, time, number of shocks supplied) (**Figure 7.15**).

Displays, controls, and options may vary slightly among different models, but all AEDs share the following components:

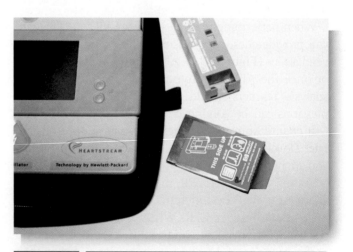

FIG 7.15 AEDs store data, including heart rhythms and shocks.

- Power on/off switch or button
- Cable and pads (electrodes)
- Hardware and software to collect and analyze data and administer defibrillation
- Guiding prompts and on-screen instructions
- Battery-operated portability

Using an AED

Once you have determined the need for the AED (unconscious guest with no pulse or normal breathing), the basic operation of all AED models follows this sequence:

1. *Turn the AED on.* Some AEDs power on by pressing an off/on button. Others power on when the AED case lid is opened. Once the power is on, the AED will quickly go through some internal checks and will then provide voice and/or screen prompts.

2. *Apply the AED.* Connect the cable to the AED. Remove the backing from the pads and place them on the guest's bare, dry chest, following the diagram on the pads. One pad is placed to the right of the breastbone just below the collarbone, above the right nipple. The second pad is placed on the left side of the chest, to the left of the nipple and above the lower rib margin (**Figure 7.16**). Maintain modesty and privacy as much as possible when exposing the chest; it is not necessary to remove clothing or undergarments if they are not in the way of the pads. Excessive chest hair may interfere with pad adhesion and electrical conduction, so you may need to shave the area where the pads are to be placed. Additionally, the chest needs to be fairly dry for the AED to function properly, so you may need to dry the chest with a towel.

3. *Let the AED analyze the heart rhythm.* Stand clear, allowing the device to gather and analyze critical data. No one should be in contact with the guest at this time.

4. *Follow the prompts, delivering shocks as indicated.* The AED will indicate if a shock needs to be delivered. No one should be in contact with the guest when shocks are administered (**Figure 7.17**).

5. *Provide CPR.* Immediately after delivering a shock, provide 2 minutes of CPR (**Figure 7.18**).

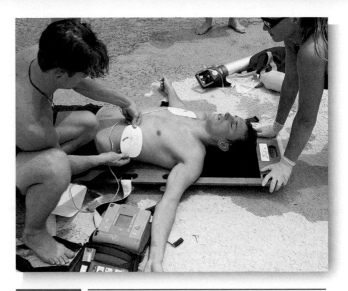

FIG 7.16 Apply electrode pads to the guest's bare chest.

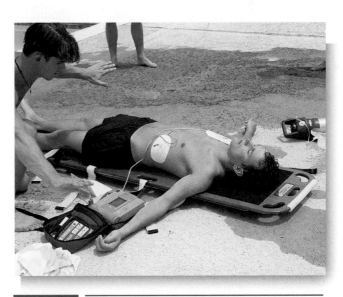

FIG 7.17 Have all rescuers stand clear before providing the shock.

CPR should also be provided following initial AED analysis, even when shock was not indicated.

6. *Provide follow-up care.* Allow the AED to reanalyze the rhythm and continue to follow the AED prompts, providing CPR after each analysis and appropriate follow-up care, until EMS personnel arrive and assume responsibility of the guest.

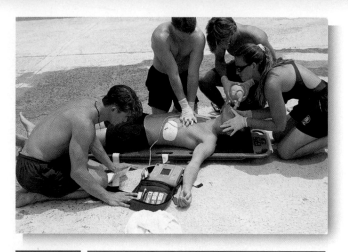

FIG 7.18 Provide 2 minutes of CPR immediately after defibrillation.

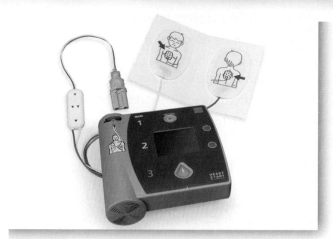

FIG 7.19 If your AED has pediatric pads, use them according to the manufacturer's instructions.

Special Considerations

There are several special situations that you should be aware of when using an AED.

Water

Because water conducts electricity, it may provide an energy pathway between the AED and the rescuer or bystanders. Guests should always be removed from freestanding water before the AED is used. Take the guest at least 6 feet away from the water and quickly dry the chest before applying the pads. The risk to the rescuers and bystanders is very low if the chest is dry and pads are secured to the chest.

Children

Cardiac arrest in children is usually caused by airway or breathing problems, rather than a primary heart problem as with adults. AEDs can deliver energy levels appropriate for children and infants. If your AED has special pediatric pads and cable, use these for children. Always refer to the AED manufacturer's guidelines for use (**Figure 7.19**).

Medication Patches

Some people wear medicinal adhesive patches (such as nitroglycerin for heart problems). Because these patches may inhibit delivery of the shock, they may need to be removed if they are blocking proper placement of the pads (**Figure 7.20**).

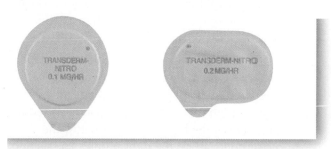

FIG 7.20 Remove any medication patches before applying AED pads.

Implanted Devices

Implanted pacemakers and defibrillators are small devices placed underneath the skin of people with certain types of known heart conditions (**Figure 7.21**). These devices can often be seen or felt when the chest is exposed. Avoid placing the pads directly over these devices whenever possible. If an implanted defibrillator is discharging, you may see the guest twitching periodically. Wait several seconds to ensure that the patient is no longer twitching before using the AED.

AED Maintenance

Periodic inspection of an AED is necessary to ensure that it has the necessary supplies and is in proper

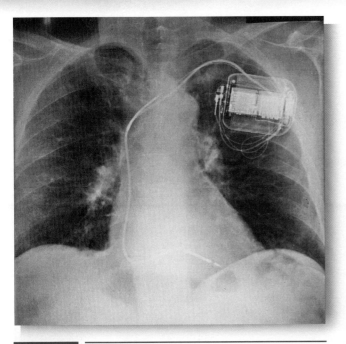

FIG 7.21 An implanted defibrillator.

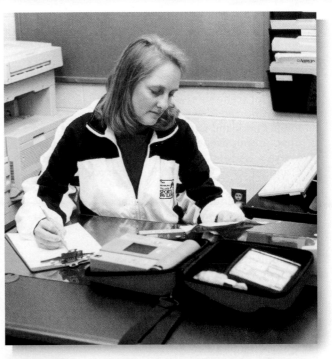

FIG 7.22 Inspect your AED to make sure it is working properly and has the necessary supplies.

working condition (**Figure 7.22**). Always follow manufacturer guidelines and maintenance requirements for your device. AEDs automatically conduct internal checks and provide visual indicators that the unit is ready and functioning properly. You do not need to turn the device on daily to check it as part of any inspection; this will just wear down the battery.

When checking the AED, verify that it includes:

- Two sets of electrode pads with expiration dates that are not expired
- Extra battery
- Razor
- Hand towel
- Safety scissors to cut away clothes if necessary to apply pads to bare chest.
- Breathing device (e.g., mask or shield)
- Medical examining gloves
- Alcohol wipes (for medication patches)

WRAP-UP

Being a professional lifeguard involves:

- Understanding when and how to perform single- and multiple-rescuer CPR

- Being able to work individually or as part of a team to provide effective CPR for adults, children, and infants
- Being able to use an AED appropriately

WHAT YOU SHOULD HAVE LEARNED

After reading this chapter and completing the related course work, you should be able to:

1. Describe when to perform CPR.
2. Demonstrate proper chest compression and rescue breathing techniques for adults, children, and infants.
3. Demonstrate how to perform two-lifeguard CPR.
4. Describe when to use an AED.
5. Demonstrate how to use an AED.
6. Describe the maintenance requirements for an AED.

AED SKILL CHECKLIST

Name _____   Date _____

	Satisfactory	Unsatisfactory
Check for scene safety	☐	☐

Initial Check and Care:

Check responsiveness and breathing. ☐ ☐
Activate EAP and get AED. (Note: If two rescuers are involved, one assesses and performs CPR while the other applies AED.) ☐ ☐
Check pulse. ☐ ☐
Provide CPR until an AED is available. ☐ ☐
- 30 chest compressions
- 2 ventilations

Defibrillation:

Turn power on. ☐ ☐
Ensure clean/dry skin surface. ☐ ☐
Connect cable. ☐ ☐
Apply pads. ☐ ☐
Stand clear while AED analyzes heart rhythms. ☐ ☐
If shock is indicated:
  a. Stand clear. ☐ ☐
  b. Deliver shock. ☐ ☐
  c. Perform 2 minutes of CPR. ☐ ☐
  d. Analyze. ☐ ☐
  e. Repeat as indicated. ☐ ☐
If no shock is indicated, provide care as needed. ☐ ☐

One-Rescuer CPR for Adults, Children, and Infants

Steps	Adults (Puberty onset and older)	Children (Prepubescent)	Infants (Approximately less than 1 year old)
Initial check	Quick check for responsiveness and obvious signs of normal breathing	Quick check for responsiveness and obvious signs of normal breathing	Quick check for responsiveness and obvious signs of normal breathing
No signs of normal breathing	Check for pulse in carotid artery for up to 10 seconds	Check for pulse in carotid artery for up to 10 seconds	Check for pulse in brachial artery for up to 10 seconds
Definite pulse found	One rescue breath every 5 seconds for 2 minutes (about 24 ventilations). Breaths should be about 1 second of sufficient volume to produce a visible chest rise. Reassess pulse	One rescue breath every 3 seconds for 2 minutes (about 40 ventilations). Breaths should be about 1 second of sufficient volume to produce a visible chest rise. Reassess pulse	One rescue breath every 3 seconds for 2 minutes (about 40 ventilations). Breaths should be about 1 second of sufficient volume to produce a visible chest rise. Reassess pulse
No pulse found (Single rescuer)	30 chest compressions followed by 2 ventilations. 2-inch compression depth. Two hands on center of chest (lower sternum, above xyphoid process). At least 100 compressions. per minute	30 chest compressions followed by 2 ventilations. Compressions at ⅓ of the depth of the chest. One or two hands on the center of the chest (lower sternum, above xyphoid process). At least 100 compressions per minute	30 chest compressions followed by 2 ventilations. Compressions at ⅓ of the depth of the chest. Two fingers below the nipple line. At least 100 compressions per minute
No pulse found (Multiple rescuers)	30 chest compressions followed by 2 ventilations for 2 minutes (about 5 cycles). Switch rescuers. 2-inch compression depth. Two hands on center of chest (lower sternum above xyphoid process). At least 100 compressions per minute	15 chest compressions followed by 2 ventilations for 2 minutes (about 8 cycles). Switch rescuers. Compressions at ⅓ of the depth of the chest. One or two hands on the center of the chest (lower sternum above xyphoid process). At least 100 compressions per minute	15 chest compressions followed by 2 ventilations for 2 minutes (about 8 cycles). Switch rescuers. Compressions at ⅓ of the depth of the chest. Two fingers below the nipple line or two-thumb encircling method. At least 100 compressions per minute
When to attach the AED age-defined pads	Immediately—When no pulse is detected and as soon as the AED is available with adult pads	Immediately—When no pulse is detected and as soon as the AED is available (pediatric pads are recommended but adult pads are acceptable)	Immediately—When no pulse is detected and as soon as the AED is available (pediatric pads are recommended but adult pads are acceptable)
Shock advised	Deliver shock. Immediately start CPR cycles, beginning with compressions, until prompted to stand clear (2 minutes determined by AED)	Deliver shock. Immediately start CPR cycles, beginning with compressions, until prompted to stand clear (2 minutes determined by AED)	Deliver shock. Immediately start CPR cycles, beginning with compressions, until prompted to stand clear (2 minutes determined by AED)
No shock advised	Immediately start CPR cycles, beginning with compressions, until prompted to stand clear (2 minutes determined by AED)	Immediately start CPR cycles, beginning with compressions, until prompted to stand clear (2 minutes determined by AED)	Immediately start CPR cycles, beginning with compressions, until prompted to stand clear (2 minutes determined by AED)

CHAPTER 7 Lifeguard Skills

PROVIDING CPR

1

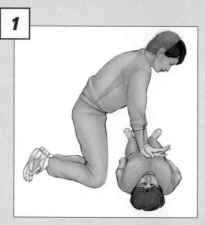
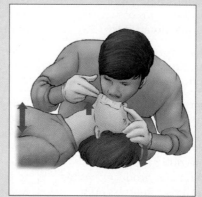

Perform CPR for an adult.

2

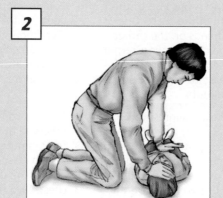
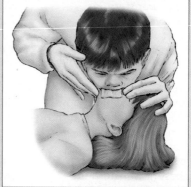

Perform CPR for a child.

3

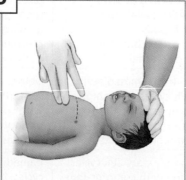
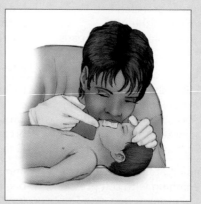

Perform CPR for an infant.

CHAPTER 7 Lifeguard Skills

USING AN AED

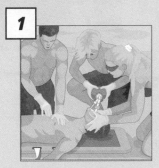

1

Perform CPR until an AED is available.

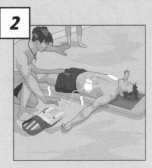

2

Turn on the AED. Attach the cable and place pads on the guest's exposed chest. Stand clear.

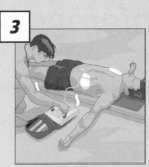

3

Administer a shock if indicated by the AED.

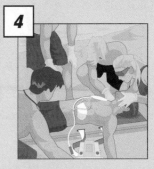

4

Perform CPR for 2 minutes (5 cycles) and then reanalyze.

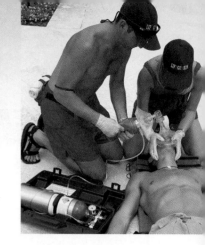

Supplemental Oxygen Support

~~~ INTRODUCTION

During a <u>submersion event</u>, oxygen supply is cut off to the body's vital organs, such as the heart, lungs, and brain. The medical benefits of supplemental oxygen in resuscitation efforts have been clearly substantiated. When providing mouth-to-mask ventilations as part of CPR, only 16 percent oxygen is exhaled by the rescuer into the nonbreathing guest. Providing supplemental oxygen support with CPR can significantly improve oxygenation of the brain, heart, and other vital organs (**Figure 8.1**). With the availability of fairly inexpensive, easily deployable oxygen delivery systems, lifeguards and others involved in a facility's emergency action plan can successfully deliver supplemental oxygen to distressed guests.

~~~ SUPPLEMENTAL OXYGEN SUPPORT (SOS) SYSTEM

ILTP™ lifeguards are trained to use a specially designed emergency supplemental oxygen support (SOS) system. This system should meet emergency oxygen requirements and also:

- Meet the specific needs of aquatic emergencies, with a continuous flow rate of 15 lpm (liters per minute)
- Maintain simplicity in use and training
- Meet the highest safety standards for an aquatic environment

You will need to understand the basic components, operation, and safety and maintenance considerations for using an SOS system (**Figure 8.2**). If your facility chooses to use an oxygen delivery system that is different from the equipment used in this training course, you must receive additional training from your facility in the use of its specific equipment.

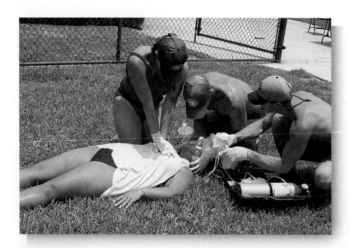

FIG 8.1 Providing supplemental oxygen during CPR.

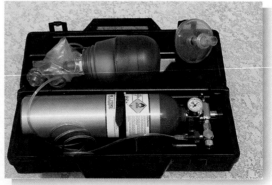

FIG 8.2 Supplemental oxygen support system.

Oxygen Regulations

Regulations for the purchase and use of supplemental oxygen vary from state to state and usually apply to the purchase of oxygen for use in non-emergency situations. An oxygen system used by lifeguards must be designed specifically for emergency use. It is the responsibility of facility management to provide oxygen systems, training, and operational protocols that meet all local, regional, and state regulations governing emergency oxygen use.

Oxygen Cylinders

Medical oxygen utilized during resuscitation efforts will be contained in a seamless steel or aluminum alloy cylinder filled to a working pressure of approximately 2000 psi (pounds per square inch). The size of the cylinder is identified by code letters. The most common sizes are D and E cylinders, which can hold 359–3029 liters of oxygen at 2000 psi and 70°F (21°C); the larger the cylinder, the more oxygen it can hold. The length of time that the oxygen in a cylinder will last depends on the size of the cylinder, the amount of oxygen in the cylinder, and the rate of oxygen flow from the cylinder. Oxygen cylinders in the United States have a distinctive green coloration and a highly visible yellow diamond indicating "oxidizer." The product label will have appropriate warnings concerning the proper handling of the cylinder. U.S. federal law requires that most common refillable oxygen cylinders be hydrostatically tested every 5 years. Hydrostatic testing checks the ability of the cylinder to withstand the pressure of holding the compressed oxygen and makes sure the cylinder is in good condition. Oxygen suppliers can provide information on how to have cylinders tested.

Oxygen cylinders have a valve that allows high-pressure gas in the tank to be delivered by a pressure regulator. The valve has three holes that allow an oxygen pressure regulator to be connected. A rubber valve seat gasket or "O" ring must be present on the top prong in order to create a leak-proof connection between the cylinder valve and the regulator. Oxygen cylinder valves also contain safety relief devices (rupture/safety disks) that are designed to safely release gas from an over-pressurized tank.

Pressure Regulator

To administer oxygen at a safe working pressure and to control the flow of oxygen, a regulator must be placed

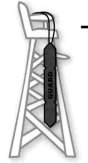

tips from the top

Oxygen cylinder valves and safety relief devices should only be removed and replaced by trained personnel using complete replacement assemblies supplied by the valve manufacturer.

on the cylinder valve. The pressure regulators used on smaller oxygen cylinders have metal prongs that engage matching holes on the cylinder valve. The "O" ring must be in place to make a leak-proof seal between the valve and regulator.

The regulator is equipped with a pressure gauge that indicates how much pressure is in the cylinder. By checking the gauge, you can see how full the tank is and estimate the amount of time for which oxygen can be delivered. The regulator also has a flowmeter that controls the amount of oxygen delivered in liters per minute (lpm). Flowmeters are able to deliver oxygen at 1–25 lpm. A continuous oxygen flow rate of 15 lpm is recommended for resuscitation efforts for nonbreathing guests.

Resuscitation Masks

There are many different models of resuscitation masks. You have already learned the importance of proper mask placement for rescue breathing (see Chapter 6). Most resuscitation masks have an oxygen inlet built in for easy attachment to an oxygen delivery system and can be used by single rescuers to supply oxygen to a distressed guest. The resuscitation mask is attached to the regulator outlet by clear plastic tubing.

CARE AND MAINTENANCE OF OXYGEN SYSTEMS

Oxygen delivery systems require little maintenance, but to ensure safe use and optimum performance, several guidelines should be followed:

• Keep the system out of the reach of children.

TABLE 8.1 *Checking Your Supplemental Oxygen Support (SOS) System*

- ☐ Important documents such as purchase receipts, receipts for refills or hydrostatic tests, and all operating manuals and instructions should be saved with the SOS system.
- ☐ Oxygen systems should be checked and the findings documented on a regular basis, following manufacturers' instructions.
- ☐ Check the amount of oxygen in the cylinder. Check the pressure gauge or the time-remaining gauge and refill or replace with a fully charged cylinder if there is less than 15 minutes of oxygen remaining.
- ☐ Check the masks and tubing. Check to see that they are attached to the resuscitation mask and the cylinder and are clean, in proper condition, and properly stored for your system.
- ☐ Check the "O" ring, regulator, and pressure gauge (if present) to make sure all parts are in proper working order. Additional "O" rings should be kept on hand in case one is damaged or missing.
- ☐ Check the cylinder for valve damage. If any is found, do not use the equipment until it has been hydrostatically tested.

- Do not expose the cylinder to temperatures above 130° F (54° C).
- Do not puncture or drop the cylinder.
- Do not allow the cylinder to rust.
- Do not use any type of grease or oil (even Vaseline or suntan oil) on any part of the cylinder.
- Do not use oxygen near a fire or open flame.
- Do not remove the valve from the oxygen cylinder.
- Have the cylinders refilled by a professional medical oxygen supplier.
- Keep the cylinder secure in a carrying case. If you must remove the cylinder from its protective case, lay it down.
- After use, clean and disinfect the resuscitation mask. One-way valves and tubing should be replaced after use.

A complete checklist for checking your SOS system is outlined in **Table 8.1**.

OXYGEN DELIVERY

Oxygen delivery equipment should be checked for full functionality at the beginning of each workday as part of a facility's opening procedures. This will allow you to respond more efficiently to aquatic emergencies. Depending upon the equipment you have, the system may or may not be left assembled at the end of each day. Refer to the manufacturer's instructions for your system. The use of supplemental oxygen should be intergrated into your EAP; this can be as simple as designating a member of the lifeguard team or supplemental responder to bring the SOS system to the rescuer.

BAG VALVE MASK (BVM)

A **bag valve mask (BVM)** is a device that allows you to ventilate a nonbreathing guest without using solely a resuscitation mask. Ventilations are provided by compressing a self-refilling bag and gently pushing air through a one-way valve attached to a mask, which is held against the guest's face. The BVM may help you feel more comfortable performing rescue breathing because it does not require you to be face to face with the guest as does a resuscitation mask. The biggest advantage of using the BVM over a resuscitation mask is its ability to provide a high concentration of oxygen when attached to supplemental oxygen with an oxygen reservoir system.

BVMs should include the following features:

- Self-refilling bag
- Non-jam valve system allowing a minimum oxygen inlet flow of 15 lpm
- Standard 15 mm/22 mm fittings
- Reservoir system for delivering high concentrations of oxygen
- Non-rebreathing valve
- Ability to perform under various environmental conditions
- Various sizes for use with children and adults

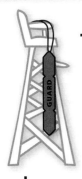

tips from the top

In order to establish a single approach for using the BVM, you can use an adult-size bag for all guests over one year of age. Avoid causing gastric distension by squeezing the bag just enough to produce visible chest rise.

It is recommended that two rescuers use the device to improve its effectiveness for rescue breathing and three rescuers when providing CPR (**Figure 8.4**). When providing rescue breathing, the first rescuer will kneel above the guest's head and is responsible for opening the airway and holding the mask on the face. The second rescuer will be positioned at the guest's side, near the head, and is responsible for compressing the bag. Both rescuers should look for an obvious chest rise with each breath provided.

A third rescuer may be needed to provide chest compressions (**Figure 8.5**). If using the BVM does not result in adequate ventilations and you suspect a problem

To reduce the length of time that it takes to set up a BVM for use, store the device so that it is readily available. Each facility will establish a system of periodic inspections to verify that the system is ready for use.

Using the BVM

Perform ventilations using a resuscitation mask until a BVM is ready for use. Verify that all BVM parts are present, including the mask, self-refilling bag, and oxygen tubing and reservoir system.

Connect the BVM to an oxygen source capable of delivering a 15 lpm flow rate. Start the flow of oxygen and allow the reservoir bag to fill completely (**Figure 8.3**).

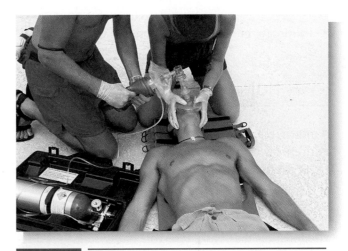

FIG 8.4   BVMs are most effective with multiple rescuers.

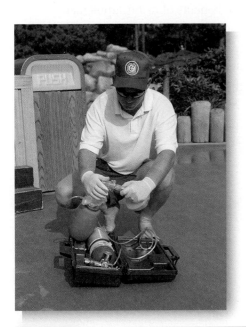

FIG 8.3   Use a BVM attached to an oxygen system.

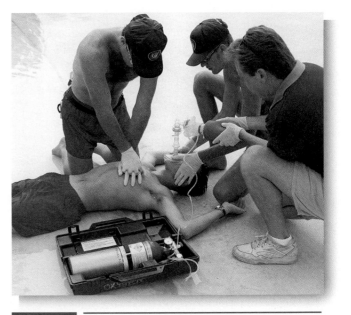

FIG 8.5   A team approach during CPR.

with the BVM, immediately return to ventilating the guest with a resuscitation mask until another BVM is available or the problem is fixed. Never delay ventilations while correcting problems with a BVM.

If you do not see an obvious chest rise during ventilation, the guest is not getting enough oxygen volume. You must attempt to correct this problem immediately. The most common problem associated with using a BVM is the inability to provide enough volume. This problem is usually caused by:

- Failure to maintain a good mask seal
- Failure to maintain an open airway
- Failure to squeeze the bag to generate the necessary volume of air
- Failure to remove a foreign body airway obstruction

NON-REBREATHING MASK

A non-rebreathing mask is the preferred method of administering oxygen in the prehospital setting to those who are breathing with difficulty or suffering from a medical condition that demands supplemental oxygen (such as a heart attack, stroke, seizure, or recent submersion event). This specialized mask is a combination mask and reservoir bag system (see **Figure 8.6**). Oxygen fills the reservoir bag, which is attached to the mask by a one-way valve. Exhaled air escapes through flapper valve ports on the sides of the mask. These valves prevent the guest from rebreathing exhaled gases, resulting in a consistently high concentration of oxygen delivery. To be effective, a non-rebreathing mask must be attached to a supplemental oxygen system capable of delivering an oxygen flow rate of 10–15 lpm. This flow rate is needed to avoid the reservoir bag collapsing during use. If your facility is using a non-rebreathing mask with its supplemental oxygen system, you will be instructed how to apply and use the mask.

WRAP-UP

Being a professional lifeguard involves:

- Understanding the need for supplemental oxygen
- Using an SOS system promptly and efficiently
- Using a BVM as part of a team approach to resuscitation

WHAT YOU SHOULD HAVE LEARNED

After reading this chapter and completing the related course work, you should be able to:

1. Explain the benefits of using supplemental oxygen during resuscitation efforts.
2. Demonstrate how to use a supplemental oxygen support system to assist resuscitation efforts.
3. Explain the safety precautions necessary when using an SOS system.
4. Explain the basic care and maintenance of an SOS system.
5. Demonstrate how to use a BVM or non-rebreathing mask to assist in supplemental oxygen delivery.

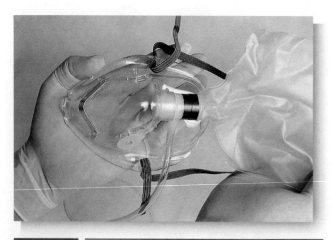

FIG 8.6   Non-rebreathing mask for a guest experiencing difficulty breathing.

CHAPTER 8 Lifeguard Skills

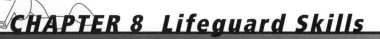

SUPPLEMENTAL OXYGEN SUPPORT (SOS) SYSTEM

1

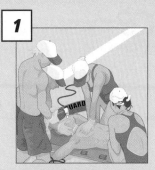

Assess the guest's condition and need for supplemental oxygen.

2

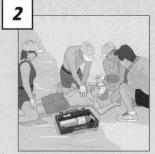

Provide supplemental oxygen through a BVM.

3

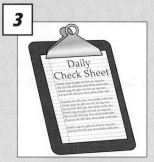

Daily Check Sheet

Properly maintain the SOS system.

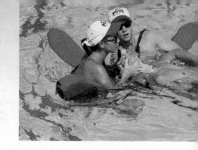

chapter

9

Guest on the Surface— Not Breathing

~~~ INTRODUCTION

This chapter introduces the skills necessary for dealing with water emergencies that require lifeguards to assist or rescue a guest on the surface who is not breathing.

~~~ REAR HUG RESCUE FOR NONBREATHING GUEST

Use the rear hug rescue when a guest is on the surface and not breathing; the guest may be floating face down on the surface in a vertical or horizontal position. When a guest is not breathing, the brain is not receiving oxygen, which can rapidly lead to irreversible brain damage. In these cases, it is important to begin resuscitation as quickly as possible. While performing the rescue and moving the guest toward the extrication point, you should begin rescue breathing in the water using a resuscitation mask.

To execute the rear hug with rescue breathing for nonbreathing guests:

1. Blow your whistle, point to the guest, hit the E-Stop (if one is present), perform a compact jump entry, and approach stroke to a position directly behind the distressed guest.

2. Extend your arms under the guest's armpits and wrap your hands around the chest to elevate the guest above the surface of the water (**Figure 9.1**). If the guest is floating at or near the surface of the water with his or her legs horizontal, swim to a position behind and almost on top of the guest; this position will

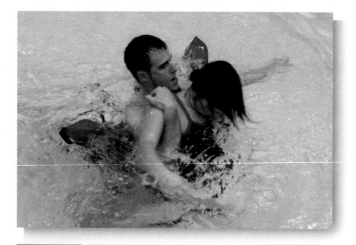

FIG 9.1 Rear hug rescue for nonbreathing guest.

make it possible for you to put your arms under the guest's armpits.

3. Pull the guest backward to remove his or her face from the water. Keep your body and head slightly to the side. Either lean in close or lean back comfortably to avoid injury should the guest snap his or her head back suddenly.

4. Pull the guest backward across the rescue tube; kick your legs to help as you pull. If the rescue tube has been placed properly, the guest's head will naturally fall back into an open airway position (**Figure 9.2**).

5. Once the guest is in an open airway position, check responsiveness, assess breathing, and begin moving the guest toward the extrication point. Once you have determined that the guest is unresponsive and not breathing, signal for assistance and any necessary equipment (e.g., backboard).

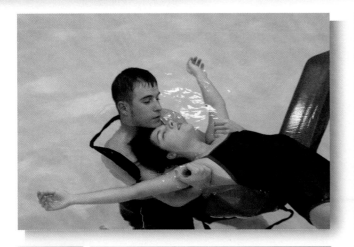

FIG 9.2   Position the guest on the rescue tube.

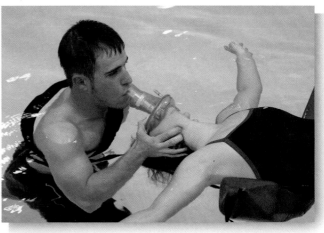

FIG 9.4   Provide rescue breathing while moving the guest toward the extrication point.

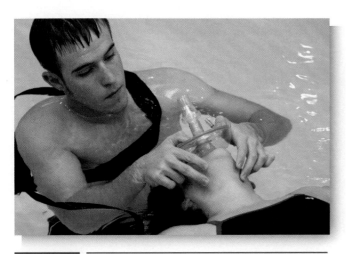

FIG 9.3   Place the resuscitation mask on the guest's face.

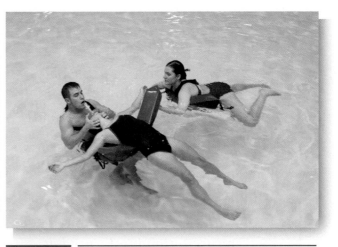

FIG 9.5   Second lifeguard assisting in the rescue.

6. Make sure the one-way valve on the resuscitation mask is attached before placing the mask over the guest's nose and mouth. Open the airway and begin rescue breathing (**Figure 9.3**).

7. To open the airway, perform the jaw-thrust with head tilt. Place your thumbs over the mask and press downward against the cheekbones. Place your index fingers under the angles of the jaw on both sides of the guest's head and lift the jaw upward as you tilt the head back.

8. Take a normal breath and blow 2 ventilations into the valve so that the chest visibly rises (**Figure 9.4**). Continue moving toward the extrication point while performing steps 5–8.

9. If assistance is available, a second lifeguard can swim alongside the guest, pulling or pushing him or her through the water (**Figure 9.5**).

RAPID EXTRICATION (REMOVAL FROM THE WATER)

Removing a nonbreathing guest from the water can be difficult and potentially dangerous. You can remove the guest quickly and safely from the water with the aid of a second lifeguard and a **backboard** (**Figure 9.6**). *This technique is used only when the guest is not breathing and does not have a suspected spinal injury.*

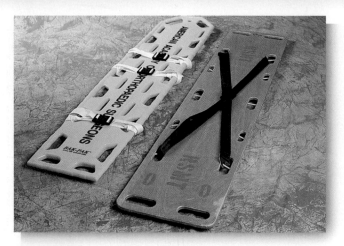

FIG 9.6 Backboard.

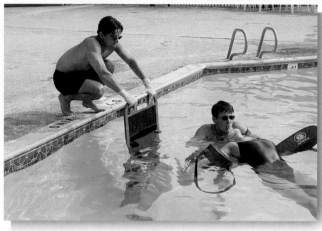

FIG 9.7 Position the backboard in the water.

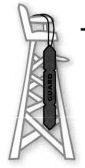

tips from the top

Frequent practice is the only method for maintaining a high level of skill competency and confidence in using a resuscitation mask for rescue breathing in the water. You must become very familiar with the specific type of resuscitation masks used at your facility.

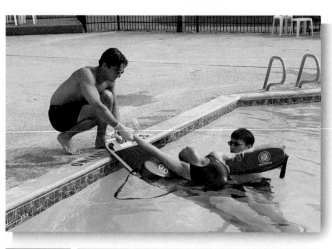

FIG 9.8 Hold the guest's arm and remove the rescue tube.

As with all rescue techniques, you must practice this skill at your facility with your lifeguard team and equipment. You should familiarize yourself with the backboard in the water and may need to modify this technique according to your facility's design. The size of the guest and the number of lifeguards available to help in the rescue may also affect the technique.

To perform **rapid extrication**:

1. The primary lifeguard moves the guest toward the side of the pool while the secondary lifeguard brings the backboard to the edge of the water and removes the head immobilizer. The secondary lifeguard places the board vertically in the water against the wall, getting the head pad of the board into the water whenever possible (**Figure 9.7**).

2. As the primary lifeguard approaches the backboard, he or she moves into position at the side of the guest and raises the guest's arm so the secondary lifeguard can grasp the wrist.

3. The primary lifeguard slides the rescue tube out from under the guest before contact is made with the backboard (**Figure 9.8**).

4. The secondary lifeguard holds the backboard with one hand and the guest's wrist with the other. The primary lifeguard is alongside the backboard, stabilizing it in the water (**Figure 9.9**).

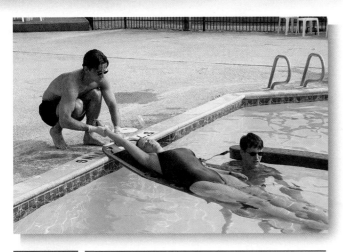

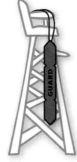

tips from the top

Do not try to lift the backboard during the rapid extrication. Instead, slide the backboard onto the deck. Use the gutter or edge as a pivot point to help. When additional lifeguards are available, they can assist by pulling or pushing the backboard.

FIG 9.9 Coordinate your efforts to place the guest on the backboard.

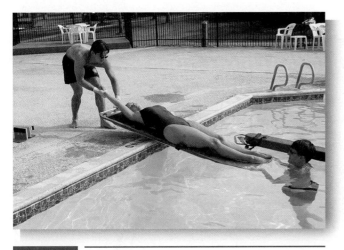

FIG 9.10 Pull and push the backboard to slide it out of the water.

5. Once the guest is positioned properly (centered on the backboard), the secondary lifeguard signals that he or she is ready to remove the guest. As the secondary lifeguard pulls the backboard onto the deck, the primary lifeguard pushes the backboard from the water (**Figure 9.10**).

6. Once the guest is on land, reassess and provide care as needed.

Special Situations

If the guest is very large or the distance from the static water line to the deck is great, you may need to modify your extrication technique. You can do this by fastening a strap around the guest's chest to secure him or her to the backboard. While the secondary lifeguard holds the guest's wrist, the primary lifeguard fastens the strap high on the guest's chest and under the guest's armpits. Once the chest strap is secured, the secondary lifeguard can release the guest's wrist.

Upon communication between the two lifeguards, the secondary lifeguard can pull the backboard with both hands while stepping backwards and sliding the backboard onto the deck. The primary lifeguard can push the backboard or climb out of the water and help the secondary lifeguard pull the backboard onto the deck.

CARING FOR THE GUEST ON LAND

Once you have moved the backboard to a level area at least 6 feet away from the water's edge, check responsiveness and assess breathing. Activate the EAP immediately, if not already done.

If the guest has a pulse but is not breathing, provide rescue breathing using a resuscitation mask or BVM attached to oxygen. If the guest does not have a pulse and is not breathing, begin CPR and communicate the need for an AED, if one is not on scene. Once the guest begins breathing, place the guest in the recovery position. Continue to provide supplemental oxygen support if necessary and monitor the guest until EMS personnel arrive.

WRAP-UP

Being a professional lifeguard involves:

- Responding quickly to an emergency
- Performing rescues for nonbreathing guests
- Working as a team to remove nonbreathing guests from the water efficiently
- Managing the guest's needs in the water and on land

WHAT YOU SHOULD HAVE LEARNED

After reading this chapter and completing the related course work, you should be able to:

1. Adapt the rear hug technique to rescue a nonbreathing guest.
2. Demonstrate how to provide care for a nonbreathing guest in the water.
3. Safely and quickly remove a nonbreathing guest from the water.
4. Reassess a guest's condition after removal from the water and provide additional care as needed.

CHAPTER 9 Lifeguard Skills

RAPID EXTRICATION OF A NONBREATHING GUEST

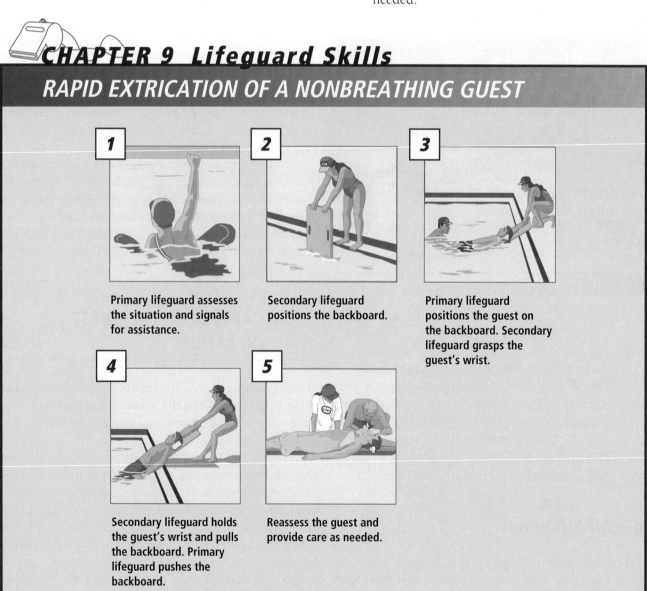

1 Primary lifeguard assesses the situation and signals for assistance.

2 Secondary lifeguard positions the backboard.

3 Primary lifeguard positions the guest on the backboard. Secondary lifeguard grasps the guest's wrist.

4 Secondary lifeguard holds the guest's wrist and pulls the backboard. Primary lifeguard pushes the backboard.

5 Reassess the guest and provide care as needed.

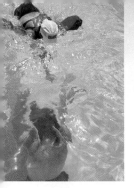

Submerged Guest

~~~ INTRODUCTION

There are times when a guest may be just a few feet under water but is still unable to get back to the surface. For example, when a guest goes off a slide, enters the water quickly, and submerges under the surface, he or she may not be able to regain footing. In this chapter, you will learn about rescues for submerged guests who are conscious and unconscious, both in and out of your reach from the water's surface.

~~~ DUCK PLUCK RESCUE

You may be able to reach a submerged guest within arm's reach without going completely underwater yourself. The **duck pluck rescue** allows you to remain on the surface of the water, with your rescue tube between you and the guest, while bringing the guest to the surface.

For Conscious Submerged Guests

1. Whistle, point to the guest, hit the E-Stop (if one is present), perform a compact jump entry, and approach the guest.
2. Stop swimming when you are slightly in front of and above the guest (**Figure 10.1**).
3. Hold your rescue tube with one hand in the middle of the tube. With the other hand, reach over the rescue tube toward the guest. You may need to submerge your head to look down into the water.

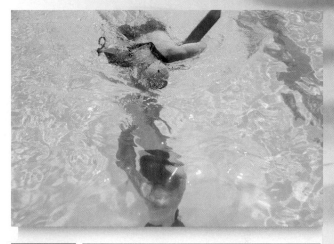

FIG 10.1 Position yourself above the guest.

4. Grab the guest's arm or hand and pull him or her to the surface (**Figure 10.2**).
5. With your hand on the rescue tube, push the tube under the guest's armpits and into the chest (similar to the front drive). Push the rescue tube with one hand while you are pulling the guest up with your other hand. This will keep you from colliding with the guest or pulling yourself over the top of your rescue tube (**Figure 10.3**).
6. Keep the arm holding the rescue tube straight and your elbow locked. Talk to the guest to calm and reassure him or her while moving toward the side of the pool or an extrication point.

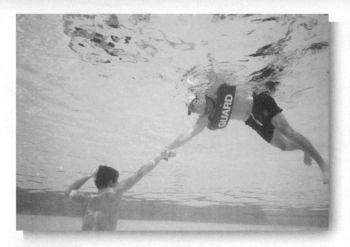

FIG 10.2   Grasp the guest's arm or hand.

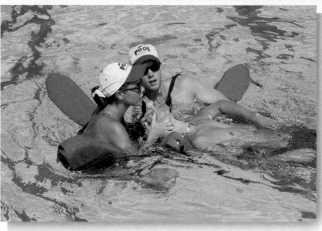

FIG 10.4   Position an unresponsive guest for rescue breathing.

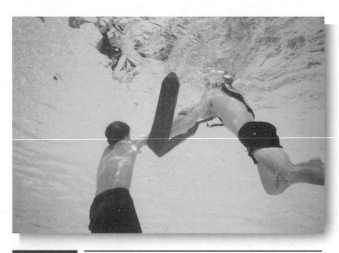

FIG 10.3   Pull the guest to the surface and position the rescue tube.

For Unconscious Submerged Guests

1. Whistle, point to the guest, hit the E-Stop (if one is present), perform a compact jump entry, and approach the guest.

2. Stop swimming when you are slightly in front of and above the guest.

3. Hold your rescue tube with one hand in the middle of the tube. With the other hand, reach over the rescue tube toward the guest. You may need to submerge your head to look down into the water.

4. Grab the guest's arm or hand and pull the guest to the surface in a face-up position.

5. Reach over the rescue tube with both hands and lock your arms under the guest's armpits. Pull the guest backward (in a rear hug position) onto the rescue tube with his or her face up (**Figure 10.4**).

6. Open the airway and assess breathing.

7. Move toward the extrication point, beginning rescue breathing if necessary.

〰 DEEP WATER RESCUE

If you cannot reach the submerged guest from the water's surface, you will need to execute a **deep water rescue**:

1. Whistle, point to the guest, hit the E-Stop (if one is present), perform a compact jump entry, and approach the guest.

2. When you are directly above the guest, stop and release the rescue tube from under your armpits. Be sure the strap is still across your chest and shoulder.

3. Execute a **feet-first surface dive** so that you come to a position directly behind the submerged guest (**Figure 10.5**).

4. With your free hand, reach across the guest's chest. If possible, move your hand up under his or her armpit (**Figure 10.6**).

5. Locate the rescue tube strap with your other hand and feed the strap into the hand across the

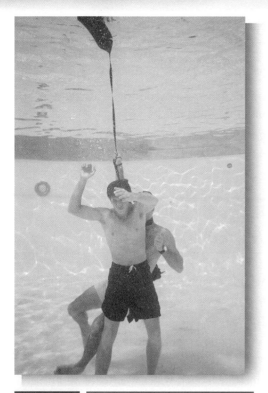

FIG 10.5 Execute a feet-first surface dive to a position behind the guest.

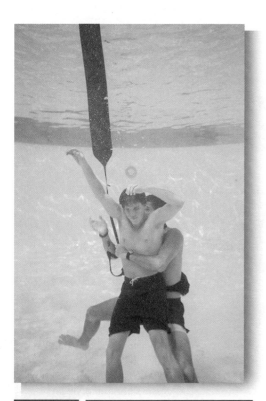

FIG 10.6 Reach across the guest's chest.

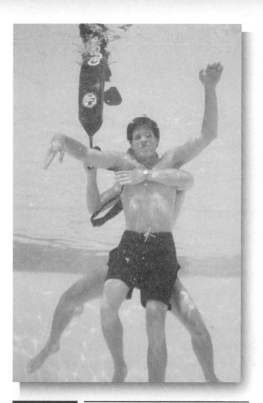

FIG 10.7 Feed the excess rope into your hand that is across the chest; the buoyancy of the tube will bring you to the surface.

guest's chest (**Figure 10.7**). Continue feeding the strap as you move toward the surface. Do not let go of the strap with both hands at any time.

6. When you reach the surface, you should be holding onto the guest and the strap with one hand. Use your other hand to position the rescue tube.

- To place the rescue tube in front of a guest, grasp it with your free hand (close to the middle of the rescue tube) and hold on to the guest while positioning the rescue tube.

- To place the rescue tube behind a guest, move your hands and arms into the rear hug position (**Figure 10.8**). This technique will provide better control of struggling guests or guests who may need immediate rescue breathing.

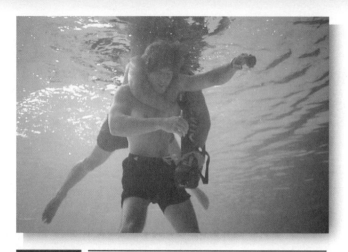

| FIG 10.8 | Move to the rear hug position for struggling or nonbreathing guests. |

7. Move to the side of the pool or an extrication point. Reassure and calm a responsive guest. Position an unresponsive nonbreathing guest over the tube to open the airway, assess breathing, and provide rescue breathing if needed while moving toward the extrication point.

≋ WRAP-UP

Being a professional lifeguard involves:

- Responding quickly and executing assists and rescues for submerged guests
- Managing a submerged guest's needs in the water, including rescue breathing if needed

≋ WHAT YOU SHOULD HAVE LEARNED

After reading this chapter and completing the related course work, you should be able to:

1. Demonstrate the duck pluck rescue for submerged guests within reach from the water's surface.
2. Demonstrate a deep water rescue for submerged guests beyond your reach at the water's surface.

CHAPTER 10 Lifeguard Skills

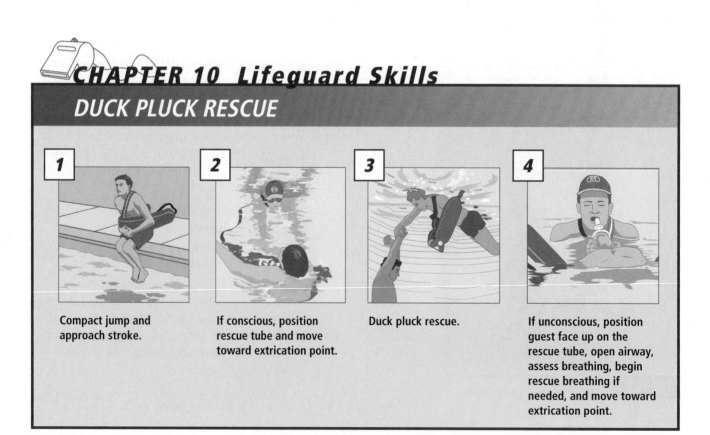

DUCK PLUCK RESCUE

1 Compact jump and approach stroke.

2 If conscious, position rescue tube and move toward extrication point.

3 Duck pluck rescue.

4 If unconscious, position guest face up on the rescue tube, open airway, assess breathing, begin rescue breathing if needed, and move toward extrication point.

CHAPTER 10 Lifeguard Skills

DEEP WATER RESCUE

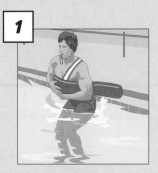

1 Compact jump and approach stroke.

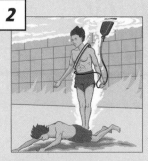

2 Perform a feet-first surface dive to a position behind the submerged guest.

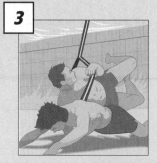

3 Reach across the chest.

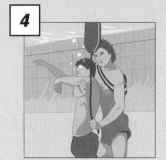

4 Feed the rescue tube strap to the other hand while surfacing.

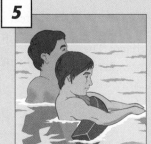

5 If conscious, position rescue tube and move toward extrication point.

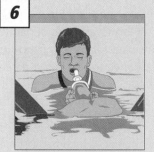

6 If unconscious, position guest face up on the rescue tube, open airway, assess breathing, begin rescue breathing if needed, and move toward extrication point.

chapter 11

Spinal Injury Management

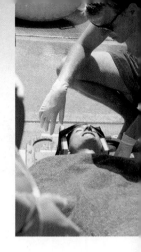

INTRODUCTION: ANATOMY OF THE SPINE

The **spine** is composed of a column of 33 **vertebrae** that extend from the base of the head to the tip of the tailbone. Vertebrae are circular or irregularly shaped heavy masses of bone and are separated by circular cushions of cartilage called **intervertebral discs**. The **spinal cord**, a collection of nerve tissue that carries messages from the brain to the rest of the body, runs through, and is protected by, the vertebrae.

The spine is divided into five regions:

- *Cervical*—neck area (which is most susceptible to injury)
- *Thoracic*—middle back area
- *Lumbar*—lower back area
- *Sacrum*—pelvic area
- *Coccyx*—tailbone (which includes the final few vertebrae)

UNDERSTANDING SPINAL INJURY

A **spinal injury** is one of the most devastating incidents that can happen at an aquatic facility. Unlike many other body parts, the spinal cord cannot be easily repaired once it is damaged, and even slight movement of one vertebra or disc can pinch or shear the spinal cord and cause permanent paralysis. Therefore, whenever a guest has suffered a serious head injury,

you must suspect spinal injury and provide care accordingly. This means restricting movement of the head and neck and minimizing all other movement as much as possible to limit further damage.

Ways that a person can injure the spinal cord in the aquatic environment include:

- Direct blows to the spine
- Head-first entries into shallow water
- Falls from a height

RECOGNIZING SPINAL INJURY

Lifeguards must be skilled in recognizing and handling spinal injuries. Always treat suspected spinal injuries seriously, and instruct the guest not to move at all. Try to determine the cause of the injury. Ask the guest or witnesses about the incident. Ask the guest how he or she feels including any pain, numbness, or loss of movement.

Signs and symptoms of spinal injury include:

- Altered level of consciousness
- Blood or bloody fluid in the ears or nose
- Deformity around the neck
- Bruising around the face, head, or neck
- Neck or back pain (with or without movement)
- Numbness, tingling, or inability to move limbs or neck normally

When these symptoms are present or the **mechanism of injury** indicates possible spinal damage, activate your facility's EAP and provide care for a suspected spinal injury.

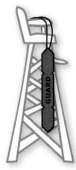

tips from the top

Analyze both the cause of the injury and signs and symptoms when considering the possibility of spinal injury.

CARING FOR SPINAL INJURY

Care for guests with suspected spinal injury requires well-planned protocols. These protocols should be developed in cooperation with local EMS authorities, aquatic facility administrators, and lifeguard staff. ILTP™ lifeguards must be thoroughly familiar with local protocols and attend frequent site-specific in-service training sessions that include EMS personnel to review these protocols and maintain competency.

Spinal injuries occurring in the aquatic environment normally involve conscious and active guests. When caring for a guest with a suspected spinal injury, enter the water carefully and slowly, trying not to disturb the surface of the water. Instead of a compact jump entry, gently ease into the pool and move toward the guest (**Figure 11.1**). However, when the injured guest is far away or in moving water, you can enter the water normally using a compact jump entry.

VISE GRIP

The **vise grip** technique is used to minimize movement, stabilizing and supporting the guest's head and neck by placing the guest's arms by his or her head. It can be used for:

- Conscious and unconscious guests
- Submerged guests and guests on the surface
- Guests who are face up or face down
- Any depth of water

For Guests on the Surface

1. Whistle, point to the guest, hit the E-Stop (if one is present), enter the water, and carefully approach the guest. In deep water, keep the rescue tube under your arms to position yourself higher in the water.

2a. For a guest who is face up, use the **overarm vise grip** to grasp the guest's arms just above the elbows at or about the ears. Then slowly move the guest's arms up alongside his or her head, pressing the arms firmly against the ears (**Figure 11.2**).

2b. For a guest who is face down, use the **underarm vise grip** to roll the guest to a face-up position. Position yourself to the side of the guest, place the guest's arms next to his or her head, and maintain firm pressure on the arms

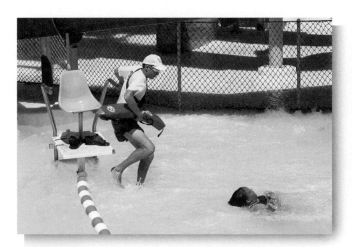

FIG 11.1 Consider the cause of the injury as you approach the guest.

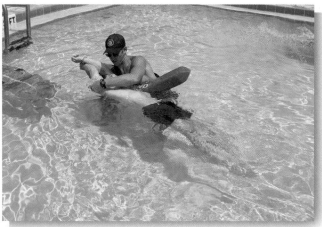

FIG 11.2 Overarm vise grip.

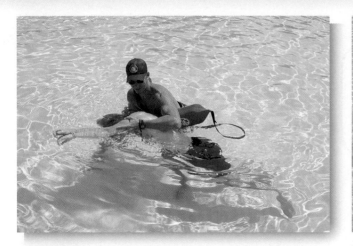

FIG 11.3 Position the arms next to the head and roll the guest face up.

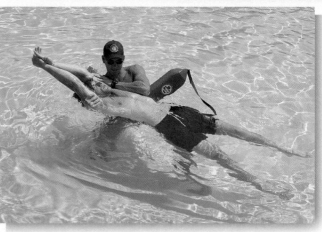

FIG 11.4 Stay low in the water and move forward while rolling the guest face up.

near the ears (**Figure 11.3**). Lower yourself into the water and roll the guest toward you. If there is room, you can move forward while you roll the guest. This forward movement will cause the guest's legs to rise slightly, which will make the roll easier (**Figure 11.4**).

3. Check the guest's responsiveness and assess breathing.

4. For an unresponsive, nonbreathing guest, begin rescue breathing, using a jaw-thrust without head tilt, while moving toward the extrication point. For a responsive guest, calmly reassure the guest while moving toward the extrication point, taking care to maintain <u>inline stabilization</u>. Prepare for backboarding (see below).

For Submerged Guests

1. Whistle, point to the guest, hit the E-Stop (if there is one), enter the water, and carefully approach the guest. Position yourself alongside and just above the guest (**Figure 11.5**). In deep water, perform a feet-first surface dive to a position alongside the guest.

2. Apply the vise grip in the same manner as described above (**Figure 11.6**).

3. Move forward, maintaining firm pressure on the guest's arms near the ears.

4. Lift the guest by his or her arms. In deep water, start toward the surface on a diagonal approach to help minimize excessive bending of the spine.

5. Roll the guest face up as you ascend to the surface (**Figure 11.7**). If you are in very shallow water, you may bring the guest to the surface first.

6. For an unresponsive, nonbreathing guest, begin rescue breathing, using a jaw-thrust without head tilt, while moving toward the extrication point. For a responsive guest, calmly reassure the guest while moving toward the extrication point and maintaining inline stabilization. Prepare for backboarding (see below).

～ BACKBOARDING

<u>Backboarding</u> is performed by two or more lifeguards to remove a guest with a suspected spinal injury from the water. For this technique, you will need a backboard, a head immobilizer, and at least three body straps used to secure the guest's chest, hips, and legs. The specific protocol you will use at your facility will be based on the equipment, staff size, and guidance from your supervisors and local EMS providers.

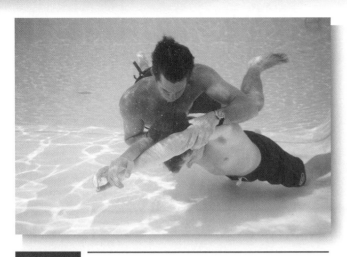

FIG 11.5 Position yourself alongside and just above the submerged guest.

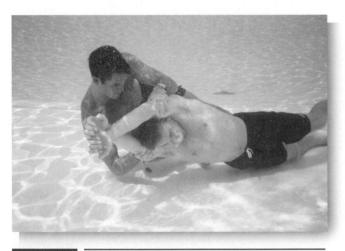

FIG 11.6 Apply the vise grip to the submerged guest.

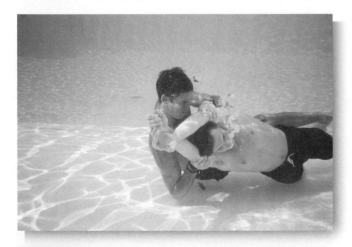

FIG 11.7 Keep the guest's head secure, move forward at a diagonal path, and roll the guest face up.

The key components for any backboarding protocol are:

- Communication between the lifeguards and guest
- Minimization of unnecessary movement to avoid further spinal injury
- Careful extrication from the water

Two-Lifeguard Backboarding

1. *Recognition and reaction*—The primary lifeguard whistles, signals the situation, points to the guest in distress, and calls for a backboard. He or she enters the water carefully, approaches the guest, applies the vise grip, assesses responsiveness and breathing, and moves the guest toward an extrication point. The secondary lifeguard clears the pool, activates the EAP, brings the backboard to the edge of the pool, removes the head immobilizer, prepares the backboard and straps, and inserts the backboard into the water at an angle (**Figure 11.8**).

2. *Preparation*—The primary lifeguard steps on the end of the backboard to ensure that it does not hit the guest (**Figure 11.9**).

3. *Placement*—The primary lifeguard follows the direction of the secondary lifeguard to place the guest on the backboard and center the guest's head on the head space (**Figure 11.10**).

4. *Transfer of control*—The secondary lifeguard grasps the guest's upper arms and presses them against the sides of the head (**Figure 11.11**). Once the secondary guard confirms control of the head, the primary lifeguard releases the guest's arms and the backboard, allowing it to rise in the water under the guest. A rescue tube can be placed under the foot end of the board to provide resistance to the edge of the deck; this will keep the backboard from sliding back into the water and off the deck edge.

5. *Breathing assessment*—The primary lifeguard assesses breathing. Rescue breathing and/or CPR should be performed on deck if necessary.

6. *Stabilization*—With the head in the appropriate position and the body centered on the board, begin to secure the straps. (**Figure 11.12**). The

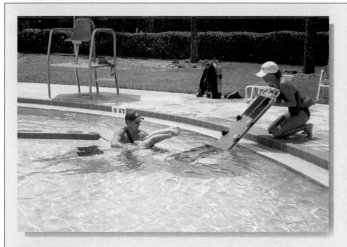

FIG 11.8 Move the guest toward the backboard.

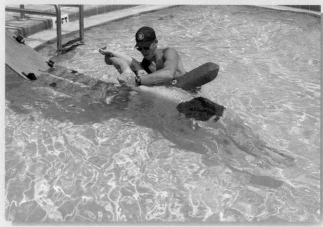

FIG 11.9 Step on the backboard.

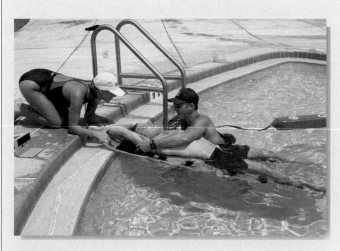

FIG 11.10 Position the guest on the backboard.

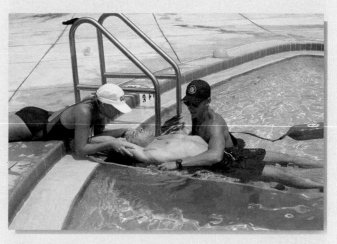

FIG 11.11 Transfer control of the guest's head.

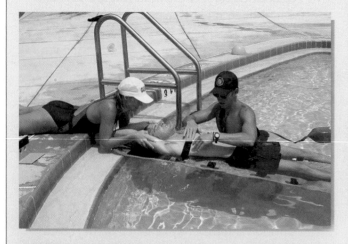

FIG 11.12 Secure the guest's body to the backboard using the straps.

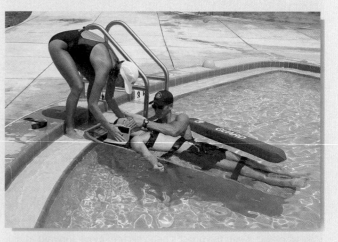

FIG 11.13 Secure the guest's head to the backboard using a head immobilizer.

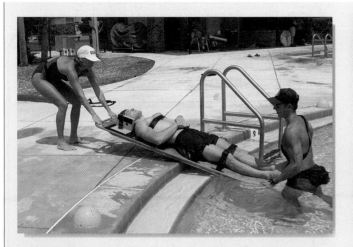

FIG 11.14 Prepare to remove the guest from the water.

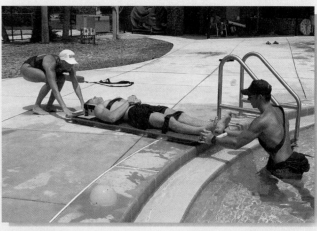

FIG 11.15 Slide the backboard onto the deck.

primary lifeguard secures the guest's body beginning with the chest strap under the armpits, then attaches the straps across the guest's hips, thighs, and lower legs (which may be necessary to provide extra support for large guests). The primary lifeguard then stabilizes the head by placing one hand under the backboard and the other on the guest's cheekbones. Once the primary lifeguard confirms control of the head, the secondary lifeguard should release the head, lower the guest's arms, and apply a head immobilizer and straps, applying even pressure on both sides of the head (**Figure 11.13**).

7. *Extrication*—The primary lifeguard moves to the foot of the backboard, removes the rescue tube (if used), and lowers it into the water. The secondary lifeguard lifts the head of the backboard onto the deck, making sure that the runners of the backboard are on the deck (**Figure 11.14**). Both lifeguards should push or pull the backboard onto the deck and move it at least 6 feet from the water's edge (**Figure 11.15**).

8. *Further care*—Monitor the guest's condition and continue to provide care until EMS personnel arrive. If the guest vomits, roll the backboard to the side. Do not attempt to turn the guest's head to clear the airway. Keep the guest warm to prevent hypothermia.

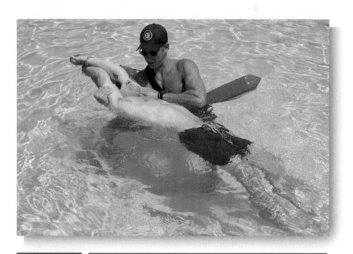

FIG 11.16 Press the guest toward your chest.

Changing Vise Grips

To place the guest on a backboard, you will need to use an overarm vise grip. If you initially used an underarm vise grip, you will need to switch the hand position you are using to support the guest's head.

To switch from an underarm to overarm vise grip:

1. Apply firm pressure with your outside hand to pull the guest toward your chest. This presses the guest's arm that is closest to you against your chest (**Figure 11.16**).

2. Release your hand that is holding the arm against your chest.

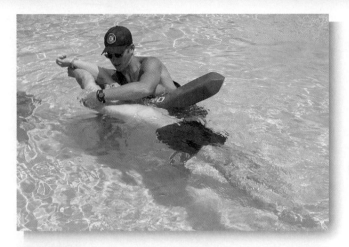

FIG 11.17 Reach over the guest and grasp the outside arm.

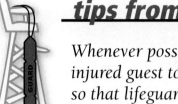

tips from the top

Whenever possible, swim the injured guest to shallow water so that lifeguards can stand while providing care. Evaluate your facility and determine the best location to perform backboarding. Consider using stable areas like steps, zero depth entries, pool ladders, or gutters to help stabilize the backboard during the process. If the procedure is being done in deep water, rescue tubes can be inserted under the backboard once it is in position. Remember that you will have to remove the rescue tubes before beginning the extrication.

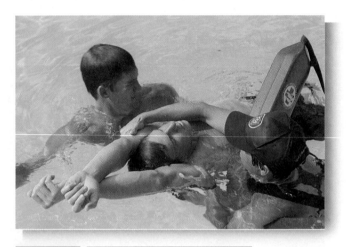

FIG 11.18 Hold the guest securely with the overarm vise grip.

3. Reach over the guest with this hand and grab the guest's outside arm, placing it next to your other hand (**Figure 11.17**).

4. Apply firm pressure against the guest's outside arm, pulling him or her toward your chest (**Figure 11.18**).

5. Release your hand that is under the guest and move it to the guest's arm that is against your chest. Continue to apply pressure on both of the guest's arms against his or her head.

Team Backboarding

When several lifeguards are available, two lifeguards should follow the basic procedure as outlined above, but should use additional lifeguards to assist with backboarding procedures (**Figure 11.19**). In this case, the primary lifeguard will help reassure the injured guest, check responsiveness, assess breathing, and communicate with the rest of the lifeguard team. The additional lifeguards should clear the area, activate the EAP, provide necessary equipment, and be ready to assist the primary lifeguard. They can also help secure the straps and assist in moving the backboard onto the deck (**Figure 11.20**).

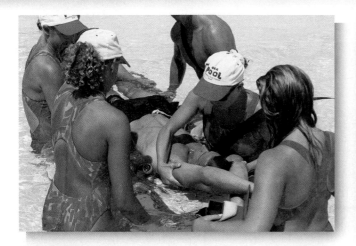

FIG 11.19 Lifeguards on both sides of the guest can position the backboard so that it is properly aligned under the guest.

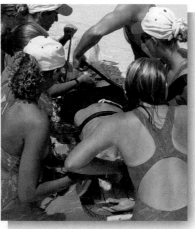

FIG 11.20 Secure the guest to the backboard.

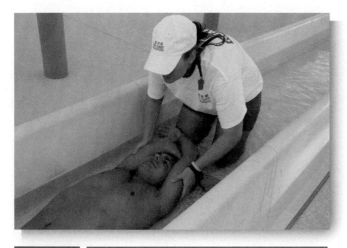

FIG 11.21 Stabilize the head and neck of the injured guest.

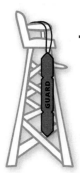

tips from the top

Communication among the lifeguards is very important during backboarding procedures to ensure proper and efficient care. Frequent practice of all team backboarding skills is necessary to ensure proper handling of suspected spinal injuries.

≈≈≈ SPECIAL SITUATIONS

Slide Run-Outs

Because of the small space available at the bottom of a slide with a run-out, spinal injury management will need several modifications. The procedure you use depends on the height of the run-out sides, the amount of room in the run-out, and other physical features of the area as well as the position of the guest and guidance from management who have consulted with local EMS personnel.

1. *Evaluate the situation*—If the guest's arms can be brought over his or her head without excessive movement of the head and neck, then the overarm vise grip can be used (**Figure 11.21**). If this is not possible, stabilize the guest's head by simply holding the head in line with his or her body.

2. *Assistance*—Additional lifeguards should position themselves along the outside of the run-out walls. The arm/hand position of the lifeguards should be spaced to provide maximum support along the length of the guest's body, from the shoulders to the feet. Logroll the guest with his or her head and neck in line with the body (**Figure 11.22**).

3. *Placement*—An additional rescuer positions the backboard, making sure that all the straps will be clear when the backboard is moved under the guest. The backboard should be aligned properly so that the head will rest on the head

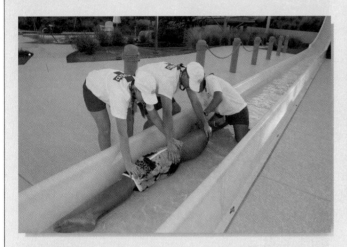

FIG 11.22 Three lifeguards work to logroll the guest.

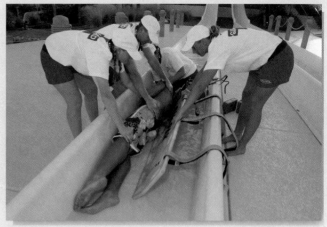

FIG 11.23 An additional lifeguard positions the backboard, and the guest is logrolled onto the board.

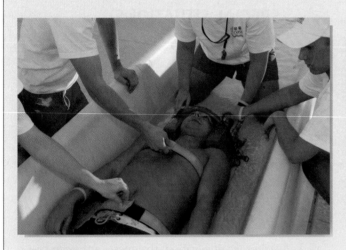

FIG 11.24 Secure the guest's body and head to the board.

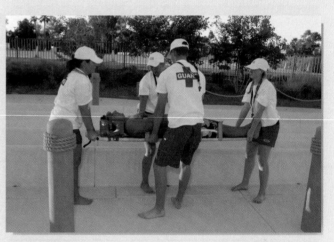

FIG 11.25 Lift and remove the guest from the slide.

immobilization pad (**Figure 11.23**). Once the guest is centered on the board, the rescue team will transition the board and guest as a unit (i.e., keeping guest contact on the board at all times) to a flat position.

4. *Stabilization*—Working as a team, secure the guest's body and then the head to the backboard (**Figure 11.24**).

5. *Removal*—On command, the lifeguards should lift the backboard together to a standing position or to a position above the side walls of the run-out. Carefully step over the sides of the slide and

place the guest on the ground (**Figure 11.25**). Provide further care as necessary.

Sitting or Standing Guest

To stabilize a standing or sitting guest with suspected spinal injury, use the **squeeze play** technique:

1. Activate the EAP and position yourself at the guest's side.

2. Place one forearm along the guest's spine and your hand against the back of the guest's head.

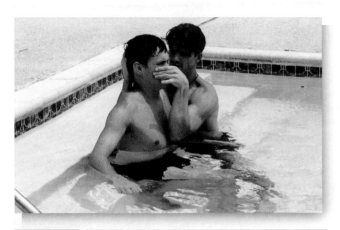

FIG 11.26 Squeeze play technique.

3. Place your other forearm along the guest's sternum and place your hand along the guest's jaw or cheekbone. Hold the head in a neutral position (**Figure 11.26**).

Rescue Breathing and CPR with Suspected Spinal Injury

If a guest with a suspected spinal injury requires res- cue breathing or CPR, two lifeguards will be needed. One lifeguard should apply the vise grip and assess breathing. A second lifeguard should check the pulse and begin rescue breathing or CPR.

If a guest is not breathing, he or she should be promptly removed from the water. In this situation, opening the airway and providing rescue breathing are the top priority. Place the guest on the backboard, but do not take the time to apply all of the straps. The team may need to apply one or more straps to provide stabilization during extrication in this situation. It is important that you perform spinal management res- cues only when circumstances indicate that these pro- tocols are warranted; otherwise, life-sustaining treat- ments may be unnecessarily delayed.

WRAP-UP

Being a professional lifeguard involves:

- Understanding and recognizing spinal injury
- Caring for guests with spinal injury
- Using techniques such as vise grip and backboarding to stabilize guests with spinal injury
- Recognizing special situations that may lead to spinal injury
- Performing rescue breathing and CPR for guests with spinal injury

WHAT YOU SHOULD HAVE LEARNED

After reading this chapter and completing the related course work, you should be able to:

1. Identify situations that could result in spinal injury.
2. Identify signs and symptoms of spinal injury.
3. Demonstrate how to stabilize a guest's head and neck.
4. Demonstrate how to use a backboard to remove a guest with a suspected spinal injury from the water.

CHAPTER 11 Lifeguard Skills

SPINAL INJURY MANAGEMENT

1

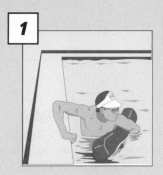

Activate the EAP and enter the water.

2

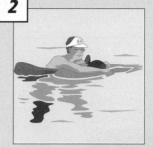

If the guest is face down, use the vise grip to place the guest's arms against his or her head.

3

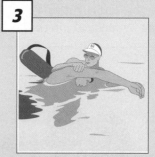

Roll the guest face up.

4

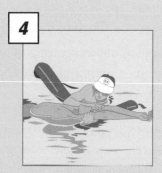

Check responsiveness and assess breathing, then move toward the extrication point.

5

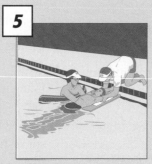

Switch to the overarm vise grip as you approach the backboard.

6

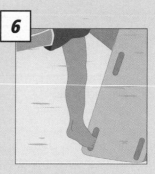

Secure the backboard with your foot.

7

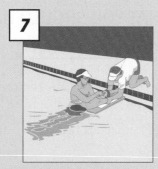

Place the guest on the backboard and transfer head stabilization to the second lifeguard.

8

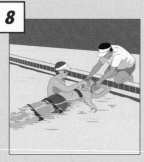

Secure the guest's body then head to the backboard.

9

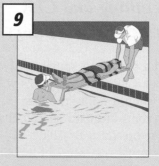

Remove the guest from the water.

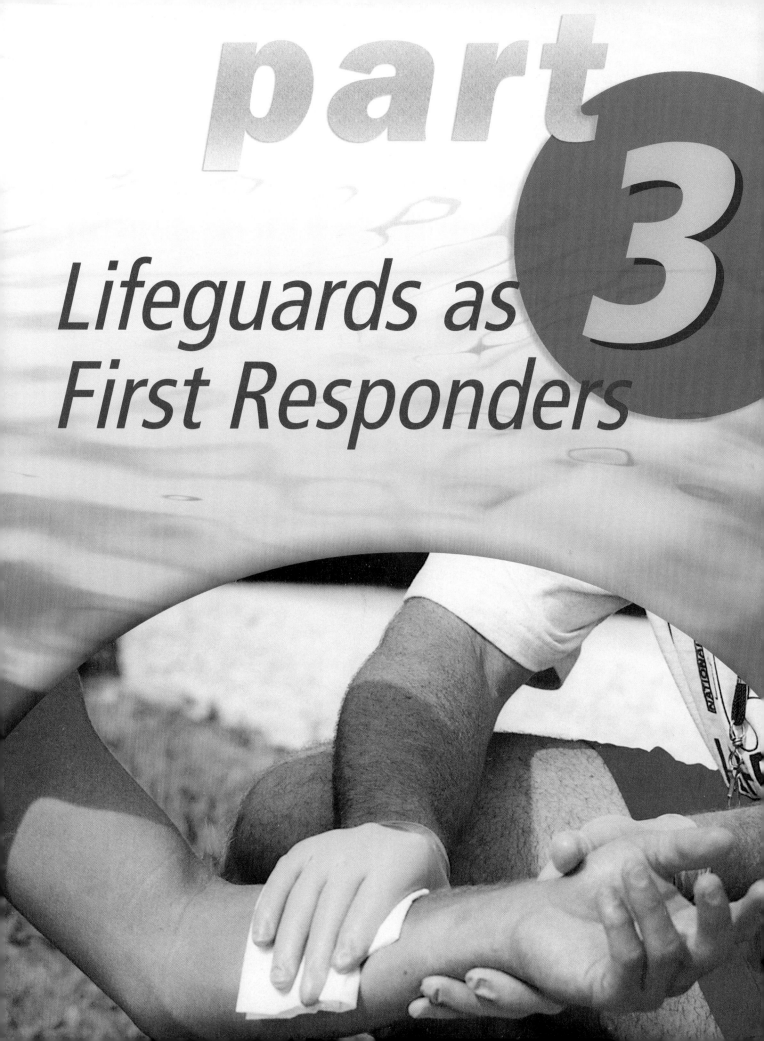

part 3

Lifeguards as First Responders

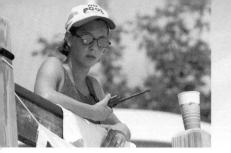

Handling Risks

~~~ INTRODUCTION

As a lifeguard, it is your job to keep others safe, and often you may put yourself at risk to do so. Part of your job as a lifeguard is to minimize these risks as much as possible by following the necessary safety precautions.

~~~ PHYSICAL HEALTH RISKS

Physical health risks may confront lifeguards on a daily basis. Luckily, most can be avoided by taking certain safety precautions (**Figure 12.1**). Many common physical health risks and safety precautions are outlined in **Table 12.1**.

~~~ PSYCHOLOGICAL AND EMOTIONAL RISKS

In addition to physical risks, you are also putting yourself at risk of experiencing events that could have a tremendous psychological and emotional impact on you, such as submersion events (**Figure 12.2**). These events may be traumatic and can have long-term effects. To minimize the emotional aftermath of traumatic experiences:

- Fill out your incident report accurately and completely.
- Reflect on the positive things you did.
- Get some exercise.
- Remember that questioning sessions with authorities are a necessary part of the process. Do not let yourself feel intimidated.
- Be prepared for media coverage that might distort some of the facts.
- Resume familiar routines such as school, work, and family time.
- Seek support from and provide support to the other members of your lifeguard team; they may be going through the same type of experience.
- Do not be afraid to ask for help. Take advantage of trained mental health professionals who can help you deal with stress after a traumatic experience.

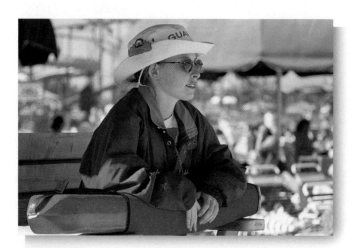

FIG 12.1 Protect yourself from physical health risks.

TABLE 12.1 *Physical Health Risks and Safety Precautions*

Risk	Safety Precautions
<u>Dehydration</u> or heat-related illness	• Drink plenty of water. • Sit or stand in the shade whenever possible. • Cool down often. • Eat small, light meals.
Eye injury	• Wear polarized ultraviolet sunglasses.
Skin damage (skin cancer, irritation, premature aging)	• Regularly lubricate your skin with moisturizer and sunscreen with SPF. • Remove wet suits immediately after work and use talcum powder.
Infectious diseases (hepatitis, HIV)	• Use body substance isolation (BSI) precautions, including gloves, eye protection, and breathing masks, and treat all bodily fluids as if they are infectious (**Figure 12.3**).
Bodily injury or submersion incident	• Attend in-service training sessions. • Regularly practice your facility's EAP. • Regularly practice your rescue techniques. • Stay in good physical condition.
Chemical burns and inhalation injury	• Follow the manufacturer's material data safety sheets (MSDS) for all pool chemicals. • Handle any pool chemicals carefully with appropriate protective equipment.
Electric shock	• Use care when using electrical equipment near the pool. • Seek safe shelter during storms.

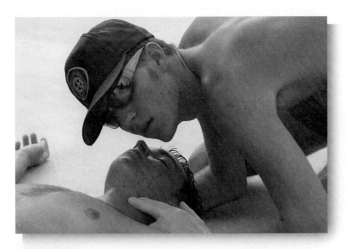

FIG 12.2 Drowning and submersion events can be emotionally traumatic.

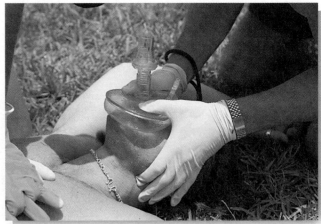

FIG 12.3 Use body substance isolation (BSI) precautions.

∼∼∼ LEGAL RISKS

There is always the possibility that you will be involved in a serious injury or fatal event. If there is a lawsuit over the incident, it is not likely to be resolved quickly. Your own involvement in the litigation could last several years and have a significant impact on your future.

People have a right to expect that they will be adequately protected by competent and attentive lifeguards while they are swimming at guarded aquatic facilities. Providing a reasonable standard of care is costly. However, the cost of not providing a reasonable standard of care is beyond measure when weighed against the lives and welfare of our guests.

As a lifeguard, you assume responsibility for guest safety and for maintaining a reasonable standard of care. You are expected to prevent injuries, perform rescues, and render care promptly and efficiently without endangering the guest, other swimmers, or yourself (**Figure 12.4**). Your performance will be measured according to the standards of care currently expected of the aquatic industry. These standards reflect the knowledge and skills expected of others working as professional lifeguards in similar positions.

Despite popular images of carefree, young, fun-in-the-sun pool guards, lifeguards are expected to be trained and capable professionals who can effectively respond to an emergency. In the case of <u>liability</u> litigation, lifeguards will be required to prove their competence and awareness at the time of the incident.

Actively maintaining the 10/20 protection standard at all times is the best way to establish an acceptable level of attentiveness in the face of questioning (**Figure 12.5**). Regular in-service training (at least 4 hours per month) will show that you are working to maintain your skills.

As a lifeguard concerned with liability risk, you must:

- Assume responsibility for guest safety.
- Assume accountability for upholding reasonable standards of care.
- Maintain your skills through regular, documented in-service training.
- Take into consideration the consequences of litigation and its impact on your future.
- Act maturely at all times.
- Accept the potential for risk to your personal safety and take proper precautions.

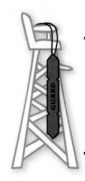

tips from the top

Being attentive, efficient, and skilled are the best safeguards against submersion events and potential lawsuits.

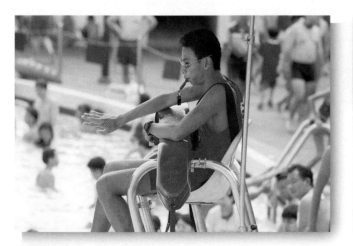

FIG 12.4 Maintaining the 10/20 protection rule is the best way to account for your level of attentiveness.

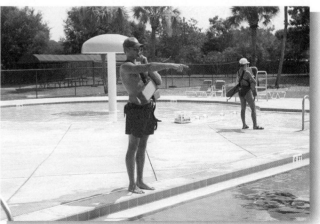

FIG 12.5 Take immediate action if you see potentially hazardous behavior.

WRAP-UP

Being a professional lifeguard involves:

- Reducing health, emotional, and legal risks
- Being attentive and acting professional at all times
- Providing corrective action promptly when needed
- Maintaining your skill level

WHAT YOU SHOULD HAVE LEARNED

After reading this chapter and completing the related course work, you should be able to:

1. Identify physical health risks you may encounter as a lifeguard and the proper safety precautions to combat those risks.
2. Identify ways to deal with the psychological and emotional impact of traumatic events.
3. Describe the concept of liability and standard of care.

CHAPTER 12 Lifeguard Skills

HANDLING RISKS

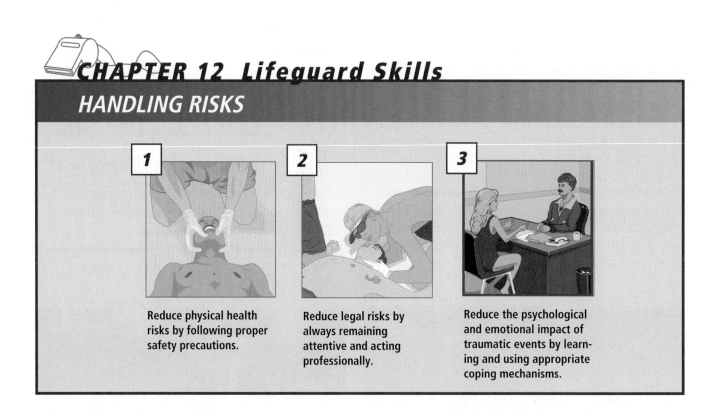

1 Reduce physical health risks by following proper safety precautions.

2 Reduce legal risks by always remaining attentive and acting professionally.

3 Reduce the psychological and emotional impact of traumatic events by learning and using appropriate coping mechanisms.

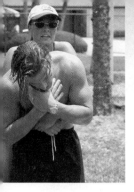

Injuries and Medical Emergencies

INTRODUCTION

As a professional lifeguard, you must be able to determine quickly when to activate the EAP and what care to provide until more advanced medical personnel arrive. Providing emergency first aid in the first few minutes following a serious incident can save lives. Each aquatic facility will have specific policies and procedures for activating the EAP, accessing EMS, and handling facility emergencies. You must become thoroughly familiar with these procedures before assuming active lifeguarding duty.

You must be able to:

- Recognize injuries and medical emergencies.
- Provide appropriate emergency care until EMS personnel arrive and assume care.
- Work as a team player in emergency situations.
- Provide EMS professionals with necessary critical information regarding an emergency event.

Additionally, you may be required to:

- Train new staff members in emergency policies and procedures.
- Develop injury prevention programs for guests and employees.
- Maintain a safe working environment.
- Document each rescue and emergency event.
- Practice first aid skills frequently.
- Purchase and maintain basic rescue and first aid equipment.
- Participate in rescue incident investigations.

ASSESSING AN EMERGENCY SCENE

The first step of reacting to an emergency is assessing the scene for safety. Ask yourself:

- Is the area safe to enter?
- Could I become ill or injured by entering?

If you believe the scene is unsafe, do not enter or allow others to enter it. Wait until the appropriate authorities determine that the area is safe. If the area is safe to enter, you should begin to look for clues that indicate what might have caused the accident. Listen to conversations and look around for anything unusual (such as a broken handrail or blood on the deck). Always take proper body substance isolation (BSI) precautions and put on necessary protective gear before contacting sick or injured guests.

LIFE-THREATENING EMERGENCIES

Primary Check

The primary check is designed to assess and treat conditions that are immediately life-threatening. These steps are the foundation for all first aid and CPR techniques you will provide. Without proper assessment skills, you may treat the most obvious or visually disturbing problem(s) while neglecting more serious or

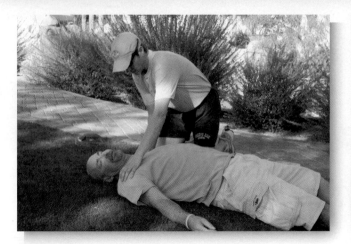

FIG 13.1 Check for responsiveness and breathing.

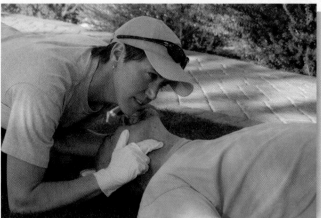

FIG 13.2 Check for a pulse.

immediately life-threatening conditions. During this stage, you will check for:

- Responsiveness
- Breathing
- Circulation

Responsiveness and Breathing

Check responsiveness by tapping the guest and shouting, "Are you okay?". At the same time, check for breathing. Look at the chest and face (**Figure 13.1**). The guest will fall into one of four categories of responsiveness:

- *Alert*—Responding appropriately
- *Verbal*—Responding to only loud verbal stimulus
- *Pain*—Responding to only painful stimulus
- *Unresponsive*—Not responding

This AVPU scale provides an easy method to categorize a guest's level of consciousness. If the guest is able to speak to you, then you know that the guest has an open airway, is breathing, and has a pulse. If the guest is not in the alert category, immediately activate your EAP.

The guest will either be breathing normally, abnormally (gasping, struggling to breathe), or not breathing.

Pulse

1. If you determine the guest is unresponsive and not breathing, check the guest's pulse for up to 10 seconds (**Figure 13.2**).

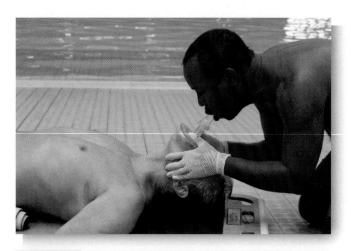

FIG 13.3 Provide rescue breathing with a resuscitation mask.

2. If there is a pulse but the guest is not breathing adequately, provide rescue breathing (**Figure 13.3**). If there is no pulse, begin CPR (see Chapter 7).

3. If you encounter a guest who is bleeding severely (e.g., blood spurting from a wound), have someone immediately apply direct pressure over the wound (using appropriate BSI precautions).

Secondary Check

After determining that there are no immediate life threats, you can do a secondary check. This check is designed to reveal conditions that are not immediately life-threatening but may require medical care. During this stage, you will check for:

- *Signs of injury*—Any conditions that you can see, feel, hear, or smell (e.g., an open wound)
- *Symptoms of illness*—Any conditions the victim feels and is able to describe (e.g., chest pain)

Perform a physical exam:
Check the body, starting at the head and ending at the toes, looking and feeling for signs of injury. Make sure to be professional when contacting the guest and focus particularly on regions of the body that may be associated with pain. Use the mnemonic *DOTS* to help you remember the signs of injury.

- Deformity
- Open wounds
- Tenderness or pain
- Swelling and discoloration

Gather information:
Communicate with the guest (or bystanders) to find out what happened. Ask what caused the injury. Ask the guest to describe any pain. You may also ask questions about the guest's medical history (e.g., heart condition, diabetes) and other necessary information. Provide the information you gather to EMS providers when they arrive.

MEDICAL EMERGENCIES

Some of the more frequent medical emergencies found in the aquatic environment include heart attack, stroke, heat emergencies, cold emergencies, fainting, seizures, shock, diabetic emergencies, asthma attacks, and poisoning. In addition to the guidelines outlined in the following sections, always make sure to follow the procedures specifically established for your aquatic facility.

Heart Attack

A heart attack occurs when the blood supply to the heart is severely reduced or stopped, and the heart muscle tissue dies. In some cases, the damage to the heart muscle is so severe that the heart stops beating, a condition known as cardiac arrest. The signs of a heart attack include chest pressure or pain that lasts for more than a few minutes, and may spread to the shoulders, neck, jaw, or arms. This is often accompanied by breathing difficulty, dizziness, sweating, nausea, and fatigue. To care for a possible heart attack:

1. Activate your EAP to summon EMS personnel.
2. Have the guest rest in the most comfortable position.
3. If the guest has a prescribed heart medication, such as nitroglycerin, assist with its use.
4. Provide 1 regular aspirin or 4 chewable aspirin if available.

Stroke

A stroke occurs when blood flow to a part of the brain is disrupted due to blocked or ruptured arteries in the brain. Signs of stroke include weakness or numbness on one side of the body, vision problems, problems speaking, dizziness or loss of balance, confusion, and sudden severe headache. To care for a guest with a possible stroke:

1. Activate your EAP to summon EMS personnel.
2. Have the guest rest in the most comfortable position. This is often on the back with head and shoulders elevated.
3. If vomiting occurs, roll the guest onto his or her side (recovery position).

Heat Emergencies

Heat emergencies can occur when a person spends too much time in a hot environment. Three types of heat emergencies are heat cramps, heat exhaustion, and heat stroke.

Signs and symptoms of heat emergencies include:

- Muscle cramps (most common in the legs and abdomen)
- Dizziness
- Nausea/vomiting
- Fatigue
- Severe headache
- Extreme thirst
- Hot skin (either wet or dry)
- Rapid pulse
- Mental confusion (including unconsciousness)
- Seizure

To care for heat emergencies:

- Have the guest stop any strenuous activity and rest in a cool location.
- Remove any heavy or restrictive clothing.
- Provide cool water or a commercial sports drink (about half a glass every 15 minutes) if the guest is alert and not nauseous.
- Have the guest gently stretch any affected muscles if heat cramps are suspected.
- Fan the victim and apply cool, wet towels or sheets.
- Place ice packs at the armpits, groin, or sides of the neck if the guest has a decreased level of consciousness.
- If the guest's condition does not improve quickly, activate your EAP to summon EMS personnel.

Cold Emergencies

When exposed to cold environments, the body may become overwhelmed. Hypothermia develops when the body's internal temperature drops to about 95°F. Hypothermia can occur rapidly as a result of cold water immersion. Signs of hypothermia include uncontrolled shivering, confusion, sluggishness, and cold skin. To care for hypothermia:

1. Move the guest out of the cold, and have the guest rest in a comfortable position.
2. Prevent further heat loss by replacing any wet clothing with dry clothing, covering the guest's head, and insulating the guest with towels or blankets wrapped over and under the guest.
3. Provide warm, sugary beverages if the guest is alert and able to swallow.
4. Seek medical care if the condition is severe (rigid muscles, lethargy, confusion).

Fainting

Fainting occurs when the flow of oxygen to the brain is temporarily disrupted. Guests may have early warning signs or symptoms of an impending fainting episode, including nausea, weakness, chills, abdominal pain, dizziness, or headache. Fainting is rarely serious and usually self-corrects after a few minutes. Guests who faint often regain consciousness quickly after lying in a horizontal position, which allows more blood and oxygen to return to the brain.

Common causes of fainting include:

- Hyperventilation (rapid breathing)
- Hypoglycemia (low blood sugar)
- Heart problems
- Dehydration
- Blood loss
- Psychological stress

To care for fainting:

- Have the guest lie down on a flat surface. If a guest has already fainted, look for signs of head and spinal injury and treat any injuries.
- Check responsiveness, breathing, and pulse.
- If the guest vomits, roll the guest into the recovery position. Use manual suction as needed.
- Loosen any restrictive clothing.
- Activate your EAP to summon EMS personnel.

Seizures

Seizures are sudden, involuntary changes in a person's brain cell activity due to a massive electrical charge. These sudden changes can cause abnormal sensations, unusual behavior, muscle rigidity, or altered levels of consciousness. These conditions occur because the brain is sending mixed signals to the muscles, telling them to contract, relax, or do both at the same time.

Common causes of seizures include:

- Drug overdose
- Hypoglycemia (low blood sugar)
- Fever
- Head injury
- Infection

To care for seizures:

- Protect the guest from injury. Move any items away that might cause injury (e.g., sharp objects).
- Roll the guest onto one side to help keep the airway clear.
- Place a thin, soft object (such as a folded towel) between the guest's head and the floor.
- Activate your EAP to summon EMS personnel.

Shock

Shock is the inadequate circulation of oxygenated blood to body tissues and is a severe condition that requires advanced medical care.

Common causes of shock include:

- Injury resulting in blood loss
- Fluid loss (from severe vomiting, diarrhea, or burns)
- Severe allergic reaction (anaphylaxis) to an offending agent, chemical, or toxin

Signs and symptoms of shock include:

- Anxiety
- Cool, pale, moist skin
- Rapid breathing or difficulty breathing
- Rapid pulse
- Weakness
- Hives, itching, and swelling

To care for shock:

- Place the guest on his or her back, as long as the guest is not having difficulty breathing. If the guest is unresponsive and vomiting, place the guest in the recovery position.
- Maintain normal body temperature. If the guest is cold, use a blanket or extra clothing.
- Provide high-flow oxygen if available.
- Determine if the guest has medication for allergic reactions and, if so, help the guest self-administer it.
- Activate your EAP to summon EMS personnel.

Diabetic Emergencies

A person with diabetes must carefully regulate blood sugar and insulin levels through a combination of medication, diet, and exercise. Any significant imbalance between blood sugar and insulin levels can result in one of two types of diabetic emergencies: hypoglycemia (low blood sugar) or hyperglycemia (high blood sugar).

Hypoglycemia occurs when the blood sugar level is too low and the insulin level is too high. It is usually caused by an overdose of insulin, failure to eat adequately, or intense exercise. Symptoms of hypoglycemia may develop rapidly. A person with

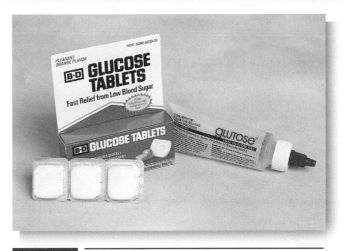

FIG 13.4 Glucose tablets and gel for diabetic emergencies.

hypoglycemia needs to get sugar into the bloodstream quickly to balance the effects of a high insulin level. A diabetic guest may have glucose tablets or gel for such an emergency (**Figure 13.4**).

Hyperglycemia occurs when the blood sugar level is too high and the insulin level is too low. Unlike hypoglycemia with its rapid onset, hyperglycemia usually takes hours or days to become a significant medical problem.

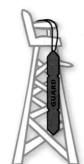

tips from the top

If you are treating a conscious guest with a medical history of diabetes, and you are not sure which type of diabetic emergency you are facing, treat the guest by providing sugar. If hypoglycemia was the cause, once you have given the sugar, the guest should quickly improve. In cases of hyperglycemia, the guest's condition will remain unchanged and the extra sugar will not be harmful.

Signs and symptoms of diabetic emergencies include:

- Diminished level of consciousness
- Weakness
- Hunger or thirst
- Vision difficulty
- Breathing difficulty
- Distinct fruity breath odor

To care for diabetic emergencies:

- For conscious guests who are able to swallow, ask them to describe any specific treatment needs and provide foods that contain sugar such as soft drinks or fruit juice.
- For unresponsive guests, activate your EAP to summon EMS personnel.

Asthma Attacks

Asthma is a chronic condition that constricts breathing passages and causes difficulty breathing. In an asthma attack, passageways to the lungs narrow and airway tissues produce excessive amounts of thick mucus. Asthma is often controlled with medication. A prolonged or severe case of asthma can become life-threatening very quickly. Asthma attacks that do not respond quickly to basic treatment are dangerous.

Common causes of asthma attacks include:

- Infections
- Excessive exercise
- Allergies
- Drug sensitivity
- Cold weather
- Second-hand smoke
- Stress

Most asthmatics know how to avoid these factors and are used to dealing with their asthma effectively. In some cases, a guest may experience his or her first bout of asthma while attending your aquatic facility and be caught completely off-guard and unprepared.

Signs and symptoms of asthma attacks include:

- Difficulty breathing
- Rapid, shallow breathing
- Coughing

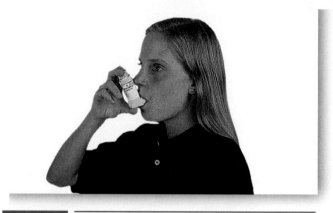

FIG 13.5 Asthmatic taking prescribed medication through inhaler.

- Whistling or high-pitched wheezing
- Fatigue

To care for asthmatic emergencies:

- Help the guest move into an upright or slightly bent forward position.
- Assist the guest in using any prescribed medications or inhalers (**Figure 13.5**).
- Provide high-flow oxygen if available.
- Activate your EAP to summon EMS personnel.

Poisoning

A poison is any substance that can cause an unintended symptom, including solids (e.g., medicine, powders), liquids (e.g., lighter fluid, furniture polish), sprays (e.g., insecticides, cleaning products), or gases (e.g., carbon monoxide, exhaust fumes).

Signs and symptoms of poisoning vary according to the substance and method of intake, but may include:

- Severe headache
- Nausea and/or vomiting
- Mouth burns
- Burning sensation in the throat or chest
- Discoloration of the lips
- Difficulty breathing
- Coughing
- Bloody spit
- Altered level of consciousness
- Dizziness

To care for poisoning by ingestion (solids or liquids):

- Suction the airway as needed.
- Place the guest in the recovery position if unresponsive and vomiting.
- Find out what type and quantity of poison was ingested and at what time.
- Contact Poison Control: 800-222-1222. Write down any information given to you and pass it on to the EMS personnel upon their arrival.
- Refer to the Material Safety Data Sheets (MSDS) for in-depth information about the hazardous materials at your facility. MSDS contain helpful information about product identification, accidental release measures, exposure control/person protection, and poisoning treatment.
- Follow the emergency care instructions provided by Poison Control. If advised, activate your EAP to summon EMS personnel.
- Provide high-flow oxygen, if available.

To care for poisoning by inhalation (sprays and gases):

- Secure the safety of the scene.
- Call Poison Control: 800-222-1222. Write down any information given to you, and give it to the EMS personnel upon their arrival.
- Follow the emergency care instructions provided by Poison Control. If advised, activate your EAP to summon EMS personnel.
- Move the guest to fresh air.
- Provide high-flow oxygen, if available.

Alcohol and Other Drug Emergencies

Poisoning caused by an overdose or abuse of medications and other substances, including alcohol, is common. Helping a guest can be difficult because the person may be belligerent or combative. The victim's condition may be quite serious, even life threatening. Although the following signs indicate alcohol intoxication or drug overdose, some can also mean injury or illness (such as a diabetic emergency) other than alcohol intoxication:

- The odor of alcohol on a person's breath or clothing
- Unsteadiness, staggering
- Confusion
- Slurred speech
- Nausea and vomiting
- Flushed face
- Drowsiness, anxious, agitation
- Hallucinations

To care for alcohol intoxication or drug overdose:

1. If the victim is responsive, check breathing and call the poison control center for advice (1-800-222-1222).
2. If the victim becomes violent, leave the area and call 9-1-1.
3. If the victim is unresponsive and breathing, roll the victim to his or her side (recovery position). Activate your EAP to summon EMS personnel.
4. If the victim is unresponsive, not breathing, and pulseless begin CPR.

INJURIES

Some of the more frequent injuries found in the aquatic environment include head and spinal injuries; muscle, bone, and joint injuries; and soft tissue injuries. In addition to the guidelines outlined below, always make sure to follow the procedures specifically established for your aquatic facility.

Head and Spinal Injuries

Head injuries include external injuries (wounds), internal injuries (damage to the skull, blood vessels, or brain), and concussions (temporary loss of brain function due to injury). Spinal injuries include neck injuries and damage to the spinal cord. When someone has a spinal injury, additional movement may damage the nerves of the spinal cord and cause paralysis. If a guest has lost consciousness, even briefly, assume the injury is serious until proven otherwise.

Signs and symptoms of head and spinal injuries include:

- Loss of consciousness
- Pain
- Tenderness
- Deformity
- Paralysis
- Bruising
- Blood from ears or nose

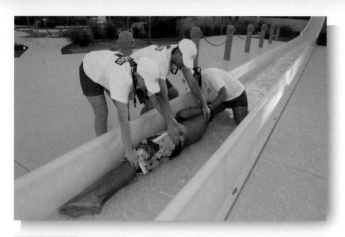

FIG 13.6   Maintain head and neck alignment while moving the guest.

To care for head and spinal injuries:

- Activate your EAP to summon EMS personnel.
- Unless proven otherwise, assume that the guest may have a spinal injury and minimize movement of the head and neck. The only instance where you should move a guest with a head or spinal injury is if the guest vomits.
- If you need to move the guest, support the head and neck as you roll the guest to one side. Maintain head and neck alignment as you roll the guest's entire body as one unit (**Figure 13.6**).
- Control any obvious bleeding.

Eye Injuries

Foreign Object in Eye

Many different types of objects can enter the eye and cause significant damage. Even a small foreign object, such as a grain of sand, can produce severe irritation. To care for a loose object in the eye:

1. Pull the upper lid over the lower lid, so that the lower lashes can brush the object off the inside of the upper lid.
2. Hold the eyelid open, and gently rinse with warm water.
3. Examine the lower lid by pulling it down gently. If you can see the object, remove it with moistened sterile gauze, clean cloth, or a moistened cotton swab.
4. Examine the underside of the upper lid by grasping the lashes of the upper lid and rolling

the lid upward over a cotton swab. If you can see the object, remove it with moistened sterile gauze or a clean cloth.

Penetrating Eye Injury

Penetrating eye injuries result when a sharp object penetrates the eyeball and is then withdrawn, or when an object remains embedded in the eye. To care for a penetrating eye injury:

1. Stabilize any long embedded object with bulky dressings or clean cloths held in place
2. Ask the guest to close the uninjured eye.
3. Activate your EAP to summon EMS personnel.

Blow to the Eye

Blows to the eye can range from an ordinary black eye to severe damage that threatens eyesight. To care for a blow to the eye:

1. Apply an ice or cold pack for about 15 minutes to reduce pain and swelling. Do not apply it directly on the eyeball or apply any pressure on the eye.
2. Seek medical care if there is pain, double vision, reduced vision, or discoloration.

Eye Avulsion

An <u>eye avulsion</u> occurs from a blow to the eye that knocks the eyeball from its socket. To care for an eye avulsion:

1. Cover the injured eye loosely with a sterile or clean moistened dressing. Do not try to push the eyeball back into the socket.
2. Protect the injured eye with a paper cup, held in place by tape.
3. Have the guest keep the uninjured eye closed.
4. Activate your EAP to summon EMS personnel.

Cut of the Eye or Lid

A cut of the eye or lid requires careful repair to restore appearance and function. To care for a cut of the eye or lid:

1. If the eyeball is cut, do not apply pressure on it. If only the eyelid is cut, apply a sterile or clean dressing with gentle pressure.
2. Have the guest keep the uninjured eye closed.
3. Activate your EAP to summon EMS personnel.

Chemicals in the Eye

Chemical burns of the eye, usually caused by an acid or alkaline solution, need immediate care. To care for a chemical in the eye:

1. Hold the eye wide open and flush with warm water for at least 20 minutes, continuously and gently. Irrigate from the nose side of the eye toward the outside to avoid flushing material into the other eye.
2. Loosely bandage both eyes with wet dressings.
3. Activate your EAP to summon EMS personnel.

Mouth Injuries

Mouth injuries can involve damage to the lips, tongue, and teeth. These injuries can cause considerable pain and anxiety.

Bitten Lip or Tongue

To care for a bitten lip or tongue:

1. Apply direct pressure.
2. Apply an ice or cold pack.
3. If the bleeding does not stop, seek medical care.

Knocked Out Tooth

To care for a knocked-out tooth:

1. Place a rolled or folded gauze pad in the socket to control bleeding.
2. Handle the tooth by the crown, not the root.
3. Get the victim to a dentist promptly so the tooth can be successfully replaced in its socket. If more serious injuries exist, seek medical care.
4. The tooth should be kept moist. Several options exist:
   - If the victim is an adult and alert, the tooth can be laid inside the lower lip, between the teeth and lip.
   - If it is not possible to place the tooth in the mouth, have the victim spit into a cup, and place the tooth in the saliva.
   - If neither of the preceding options are possible, the tooth can be placed in milk, a saltwater solution (teaspoon salt in 1 quart of water), or normal water.

Muscle, Bone, and Joint Injuries

Muscle, bone, and joint injuries are rarely life-threatening. Often, the best thing you can do is to help reduce the anxiety that guests commonly experience and keep the guest from moving the injured area. Symptoms of muscle, bone, and joint injuries are similar, which may make it difficult to determine the extent of the injury.

Signs and symptoms of muscle, bone, and joint injuries include:

- Deformity of a body part
- Tenderness or pain
- Crepitus (bone ends grating)
- Swelling
- Bruising or discoloration
- Exposed bone ends (**Figure 13.7**)
- Inability to move or use the affected area

To care for a bone injury, such as a possible fracture:

1. Allow the guest to support the injured area in the most comfortable position.
2. Stabilize the injured part to prevent movement.
   - If emergency medical services (EMS) will arrive soon, stabilize the injured part with your hands until they arrive.
   - If EMS will be delayed, or if you are taking the victim to medical care, stabilize the injured part with a splint.
3. If the injury is an open fracture, do not push on any protruding bone. Cover the wound and exposed bone with a dressing.
4. Apply an ice or cold pack if possible to help reduce the swelling and pain.

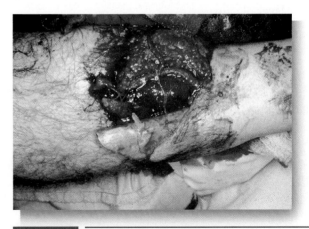

FIG 13.7 Open fracture of the lower leg.

5. Activate your EAP to summon EMS personnel for any open fractures or large bone fractures (such as the thigh) or when transporting the victim would be difficult or would aggravate the injury.

Splints are devices used to help stabilize a bone or joint injury. Splinting helps reduce pain and prevent further damage to muscles, nerves, and blood vessels. There are several different types of splints:

- Rigid (e.g., a board) (**Figure 13.8**)
- Soft (e.g., a rolled towel) (**Figure 13.9**)
- Anatomical (self) (**Figure 13.10**)

Soft Tissue Injuries

Soft tissue injuries include bruises, <u>abrasions</u> (e.g., skinned knee), and wounds. These injuries are generally not life-threatening, though they may be bloody or painful.

When caring for an open wound, you must control any bleeding and reduce the chance of infection. Be sure to use proper BSI precautions prior to any contact with the guest.

Signs and symptoms of soft tissue injuries include:

- External bleeding
- Internal bleeding (bruising)
- Burns

To care for soft tissue injuries:

- Take standard safety precautions and use protective gloves before contacting the guest.
- Place a gauze pad over the open wound and apply pressure.
- If bleeding continues and the gauze becomes soaked, apply additional gauze. Do not remove the first layer of gauze.
- Use a gauze roll to bandage the wound. This will maintain pressure and keep the wound clean.
- Activate your EAP to summon EMS personnel if bleeding is severe or cannot be controlled.
- If the wound includes an embedded object, leave the object in place. Stabilize the object by using both of your gloved hands until EMS personnel arrive and decide the best method of stabilization and transportation.
- If the soft tissue injury involves an amputated part (e.g., piece of a toe), pick it up with a gauze pad, place it in a container such as a plastic bag, and keep the part cool and dry. EMS personnel will transport the amputated part with the guest to the hospital (**Figure 13.11**).

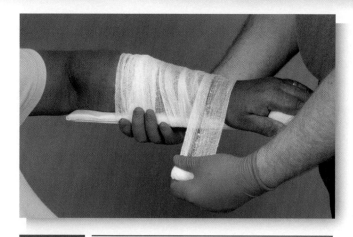

FIG 13.8   Rigid splint.

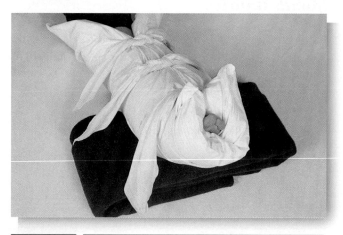

FIG 13.9   Soft splint.

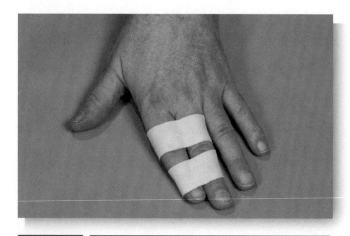

FIG 13.10   Anatomical (self) splint.

Nosebleeds

Nosebleeds are fairly common, especially in crowded places. At aquatic facilities, guests often suffer nosebleeds when they bump into each other.

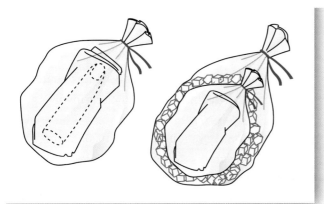

FIG 13.11 Care for an amputated part.

To care for nosebleeds:

- Have the guest sit down and lean slightly forward.
- Have the guest pinch the nostrils together at the bridge of his or her nose for 5 to 10 minutes.
- Activate your EAP to summon EMS personnel if the bleeding cannot be controlled or if the guest has an associated medical condition (e.g., hypertension).

Burns

There are several different types of burns. Thermal burns are caused by contact with heat, such as flames, steam, or hot liquids. Chemical burns are caused by exposure to dry, liquid, or chemical gases. Burns also may be caused by exposure to radiation, sun, or electricity (e.g., lightning, electrical outlets, or power supply lines). Burns are classified according to the extent of tissue damage (first-, second-, and third-degree). Burn victims may suffer all three levels of severity during the same incident. If you encounter this situation, treat the area according to the highest level of severity.

Signs and symptoms of burns include:

- *First-degree (superficial) burns*—These burns affect the outer layers of skin, usually turning the skin red and causing slight swelling. If these burns cover a large portion of a guest's body, the guest should seek medical attention (**Figure 13.12**).

- *Second-degree (partial-thickness) burns*—These burns damage deeper layers of skin, causing blisters to form on the skin's surface. These blisters vary in size, and a single blister can sometimes cover a large area of tissue (**Figure 13.13**).

- *Third-degree (full-thickness) burns*—These burns damage all layers of the skin and underlying tissue. They can be

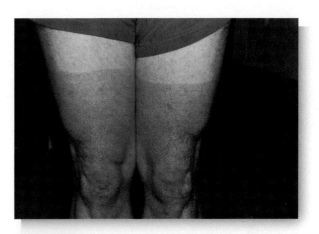

FIG 13.12 First-degree (superficial) burn.

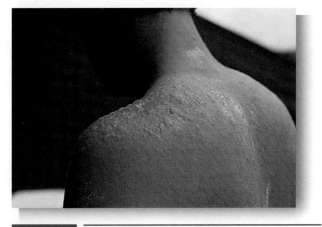

FIG 13.13 Second-degree (partial thickness) burn.

multi-colored (black, red, gray, white) and cause little or no pain (which is a result of damage to local nerve endings). A guest may experience pain in the areas surrounding a third-degree burn (**Figure 13.14**).

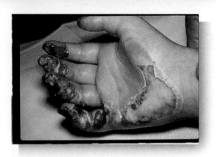

FIG 13.14 Third-degree (full thickness) burn.

To care for burns:

- Cool first- and second-degree burns with cool water, but leave third-degree burns dry.
- Remove any jewelry or smoldering clothing.
- Do not apply pressure if blisters are present.
- For second- and third-degree burns, cover the burn loosely with a dry, nonstick gauze pad and bandage loosely.
- Activate your EAP to summon EMS personnel for guests with chemical burns, electrical burns, or serious thermal burns.
- If the burn is electrical, and the guest is pulseless, begin CPR and get an AED.
- If the burn is from a wet chemical, flush it with a large, continuous flow of water. If the chemical is a dry powder, brush the powder from the skin before flushing.

WRAP-UP

Being a professional lifeguard involves:

- Assessing and caring for life-threatening conditions
- Staying calm in emergency situations involving sudden illnesses and injuries
- Using BSI safety precautions when contacting guests
- Maintaining your skill level to manage injury and illness

WHAT YOU SHOULD HAVE LEARNED

After reading this chapter and completing the related course work, you should be able to:

1. Explain your role as a lifeguard first responder.
2. Demonstrate how to assess an ill or injured guest.
3. Recognize the signs, symptoms, and causes of emergencies you are likely to encounter in an aquatic environment.
4. Describe how to provide care for emergencies until EMS personnel arrive.

CHAPTER 13 *Lifeguard Skills*

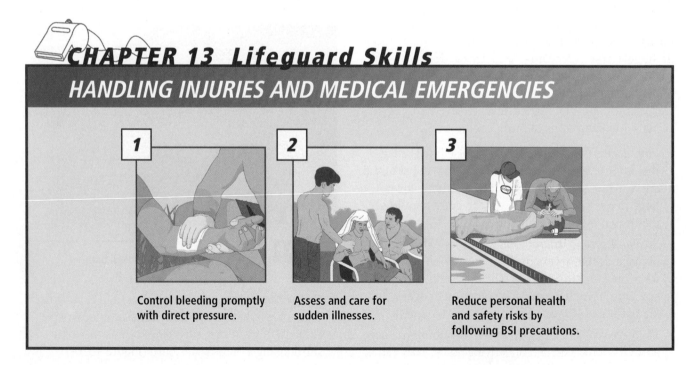

HANDLING INJURIES AND MEDICAL EMERGENCIES

1 Control bleeding promptly with direct pressure.

2 Assess and care for sudden illnesses.

3 Reduce personal health and safety risks by following BSI precautions.

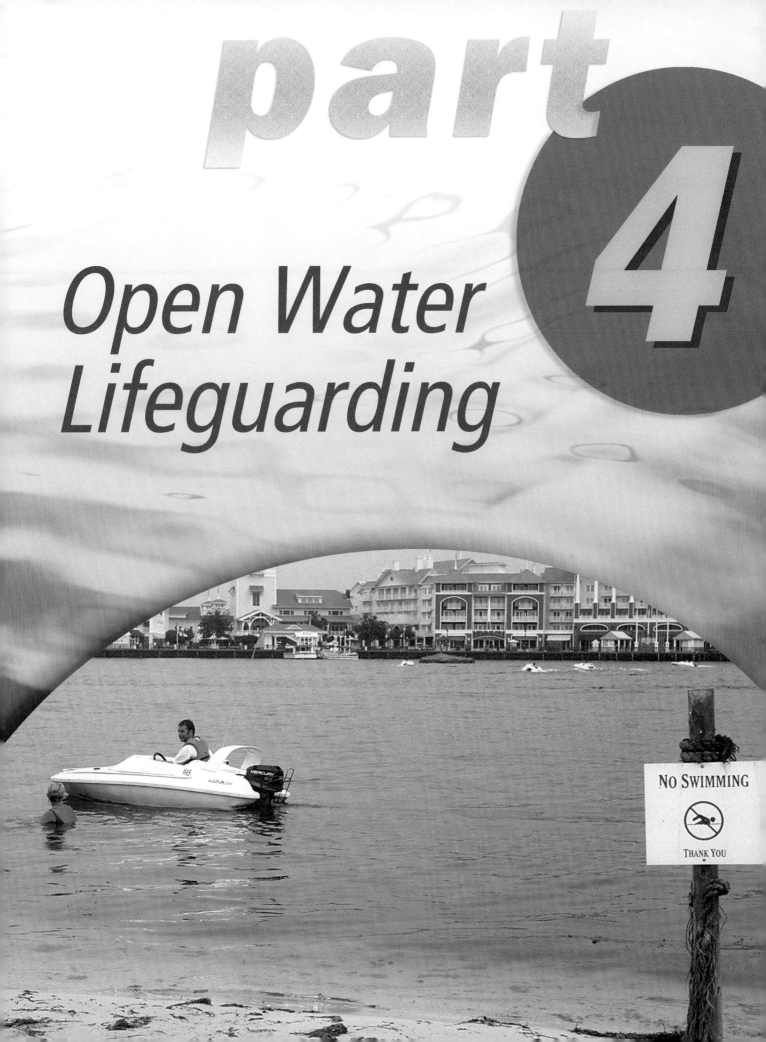

part 4

Open Water Lifeguarding

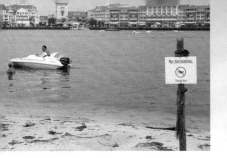

Open Water Lifeguarding

~~~ INTRODUCTION

The skills you learned in previous chapters of this text apply to both pool and open water settings; however, there are instances in the open water environment when you will need to modify your technique, use slightly different equipment, or get additional site-specific training.

~~~ 10/3 PROTECTION STANDARD

One of the largest differences between lifeguarding open water areas and pools is the modification of the 10/20 protection standard. Because Zone of Protection areas are often larger in the open water environment and have increased turbidity and poorer visibility, lifeguards should follow the __10/3 protection standard__ in open water facilities. This means that while scanning a Zone of Protection area, the lifeguard has 10 seconds to complete the scan and recognize that a guest is in distress. Upon recognition, the lifeguard should immediately activate the EAP and begin rescue efforts appropriate for the type of distressed guest. Rescues should be performed as quickly as possible. Should a guest in distress become submerged, the lifeguard (or lifeguard team) should complete a bottom search of the entire Zone of Protection area and ultimately recover the guest within 3 minutes.

~~~ DESIGNATED SWIMMING AREAS

Swimming areas and the lifeguard zones within them must be established so that lifeguards can maintain the 10/3 protection standard. Swimming areas can be delineated using buoy lines (**Figure 14.1**), floats, or flags (**Figure 14.2**). The location of these markers will depend on factors such as the swimming ability of the lifeguards, water depth and clarity, availability of watercraft (e.g., rescue boards and kayaks) for rescues, and other facility-specific factors. Swimming areas should be designated so that the entire bottom of a designated Zone of Protection area can be searched within 3 minutes.

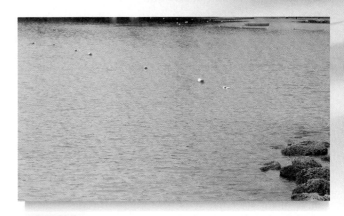

FIG 14.1   Swimming area designated by buoy lines.

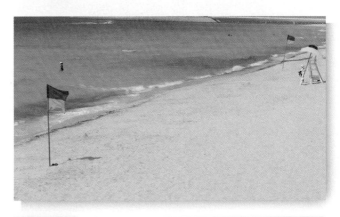

FIG 14.2   Swimming area designated by flags.

~~~ POTENTIAL HAZARDS

Open water facilities have many more potential hazards than controlled pool environments. These include waves, rip currents, tides, water temperature, water visibility, bottom conditions, refuse, contaminants, wildlife, and parasites. Water conditions can fluctuate quickly, ranging from calm water to large waves within a short span of time. As an open water lifeguard, you must be vigilant to ensure that you maintain sight of the swimmers in your zone. If you decide that the conditions are too dangerous to swim, notify your supervisor immediately.

Waves and Rip Currents

Oceanfront lifeguards must recognize that breaking waves can cause distress for swimmers; the bigger the waves, the greater the possibility of rip currents. As each wave breaks on the shoreline, the deposited water needs to find a way back out to sea. When the outgoing water cannot find a way out to sea, it moves sand away from the bottom to create a channel for its return. This can create a rip current where water will rush out to the sea (**Figure 14.3**).

A rip current will not create an undertow, but a person caught in a rip will be pulled away from the beach. Even the best swimmers can tire trying to swim against this current. Although a rip current is strong, it is generally not very wide. If you observe a guest caught in a rip current, you should assist him or her by swimming with the current beyond the breaking waves and then swimming parallel to the beach until the current is no longer present. If a rip

current is observed, swimmers should be alerted to stay clear of the danger.

Rip currents can be identified by the following characteristics:

- A channel of discolored water (caused by the sand moved off the bottom of the sea where the rip is running away from the shore) (**Figure 14.4**)
- An area or channel where there are no waves breaking while waves are breaking on either side of the channel
- Sticks and other debris floating out to sea in the rip

Tides

On a daily basis, oceanfront lifeguards need to be aware of two tides:

- *Incoming*—Reaches high tide when seawater reaches its highest point on the beach
- *Outgoing*—Reaches low tide when seawater is at its lowest point on the beach

It takes 6 hours for a tide to go from high to low and another 6 hours from low to high. During a typical day, an oceanfront lifeguard is likely to encounter each of these tide changes. Lifeguards should be aware of tidal changes during their shifts, because this can change the characteristics and safety of zones dramatically. When the moon is in its new or full phase, the tidal difference is even more exaggerated.

Water Temperature

Water may be warm on the surface but much colder at greater depths. Water is usually colder in early

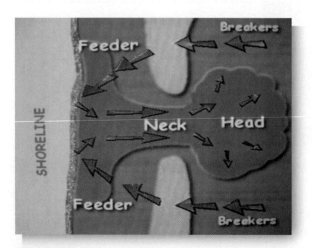

FIG 14.3 Rip current.

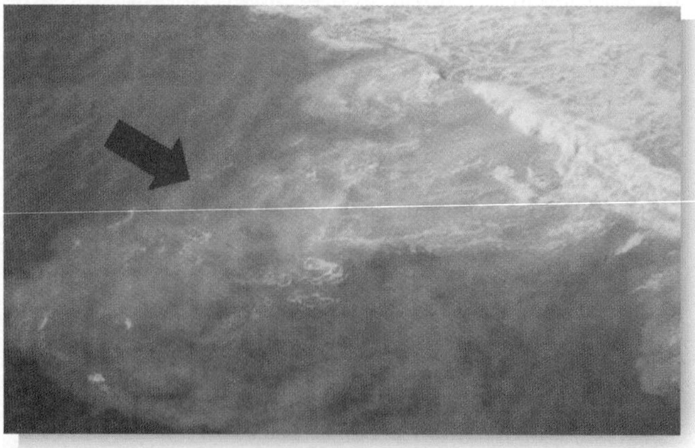

FIG 14.4 Channel of discolored water indicating a rip current.

summer than late summer. You can help swimmers avoid **hypothermia** by advising them of cold water conditions. Cold water can also complicate a rescue attempt, so lifeguards may wear wet suits while guarding to minimize the effects of the cold water during a rescue.

Water Visibility

Water visibility is one of the most significant differences between open water and pool lifeguarding. In calm open water areas, visibility is often best in the early morning. Stirred-up sediment from guests or high winds, heavy rain, waves, and plant growth can cause poor visibility (**Figure 14.5**).

Bottom Conditions

Items such as rocks, glass, fishing line or hooks, and heavy plant growth all contribute to bottom conditions that create hazards for swimmers and lifeguards. These should be removed from the area whenever possible. Many lakes have natural conditions that cause silt to build up, in some cases several feet deep. Silty lake or ocean bottoms are dangerous because they hinder search and rescue efforts.

Refuse and Contaminants

In some open water areas, lifeguards are responsible for clearing the beach of trash and debris. It is important to keep the beach clean so that animals and water fowl will be less attracted to the beach. Nearby roadway, storm, and drain runoff during heavy storms is potentially dangerous because of contaminants that can be deposited on the beach and in the water.

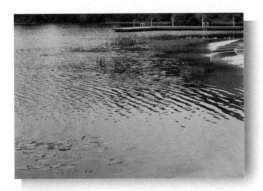

FIG 14.5 Plant growth can cause poor visibility.

Wildlife and Parasites

If there is a large population of water fowl, lily pads, milfoil, or algae on an open water area, the possibility of parasites exists. These parasites can cause skin irritation. Many lake areas have adopted policies that prohibit feeding ducks and geese so that the birds will leave the area and limit problems for swimmers.

In ocean- and lagoon-front environments, there is also potential for dangerous marine wildlife such as jellyfish, stingrays, and sharks. If marine predators are sighted, the area should be evacuated as quickly and calmly as possible. Lifeguards should carefully monitor the area and can reopen the area 30 minutes after the predator has left. If the predator returns, then the area should be closed for the remainder of the day.

WEATHER CONDITIONS

Weather conditions are a day-to-day concern for open water facilities. Each facility should have a comprehensive plan for monitoring changing weather conditions and alerting lifeguards and guests. If conditions become unsafe to swim, the area should be evacuated and closed until it is safe to reopen.

Thunder and Lightning

Thunderstorms and accompanying lightning strikes can be unpredictable and may cause swimming conditions to become dangerous very quickly. Lifeguards are often responsible for monitoring weather conditions and guiding guests to safety. This can be done both by scanning the sky occasionally for impending thunderstorms and by utilizing a local hazardous weather warning system.

Wind

High winds can result in larger waves than normal, which increase the chance of hypothermia, swimmer fatigue, and change in the normal current. Any of these conditions may affect your ability to reach a distressed guest. Two types of wind can affect the surface of the water:

- *Onshore wind*—Blows predominantly from sea to land, and can cause the surface of the sea to be choppy, especially the harder it blows

- *Offshore wind*—Blows predominantly from land to sea, and can cause the surface of the sea to be flat

Rain and Fog

At some open water facilities, heavy rain or fog may obscure buoy markers and cause swimmers to venture beyond the swimming area. Rain or fog may also jeopardize your ability to scan your zone effectively.

FACILITY SAFETY

As a proactive lifeguard, you must constantly scan your zone to prevent incidents from occurring needlessly. In an open water environment, you must take several additional proactive steps to ensure your guests' safety:

- Develop an awareness of the activities outside your lifeguard zone that may affect the safety of guests in your zone.
- Caution swimmers about the dangers of swimming beyond the swimming area.
- Warn guests not to swim in unguarded or restricted areas.
- Enforce the safety rules of your facility.
- Inform rule violators of the actions you or your supervisor will take on behalf of your facility if they continue to disregard the rules.

Each facility should conduct frequent and regular safety inspections of both the immediate area (beach, shoreline, and shallow water) and equipment. While conducting your inspection, carefully survey the entire area for sharp or potentially dangerous objects:

- Broken glass, rocks, litter, etc.
- Any objects near lifeguard stands that could cause potential injury as guards come down from the stands
- Loose rocks, loose or rotting wood, and weak or frayed anchor lines on docks, jetties, or breakers
- Depressions and obstructions in shallow water

Inspect your equipment daily for cleanliness, condition, and location. Always report any damaged or missing equipment to your supervisor immediately.

CHAIN OF COMMAND

Open water facilities will have one or more supervisors. There may be several people in the chain of command including aquatic coordinator, facility supervisor, head lifeguard, park ranger, security guard, and swimming and boating instructors. As with pool facilities, you must be thoroughly familiar with the personnel in your chain of command. In an emergency, it will be critical for you to know whom to contact.

EMERGENCY RESPONSE

In emergency situations, you will need to understand your role and be ready to respond appropriately. Know your facility's EAP, the location of emergency equipment, and the layout of the waterfront.

POLICIES AND PROCEDURES

Each waterfront facility will have its own policies and procedures for opening and closing, ensuring water safety, responding to emergencies, and maintaining beach security. These policies and procedures should list responsibilities of various personnel. Your facility-specific training should include each lifeguard's responsibilities and reporting procedures. The development of risk management and accident prevention plans are management's responsibility, but each lifeguard must know his or her individual duties and responsibilities for the supervision of swimmers and enforcement of the facility's rules.

WATERCRAFT

If your waterfront facility uses watercraft for rescues, it will be important for you to learn how to use them correctly in various rescue situations and in risky weather conditions. Practice until your skill level meets your facility's standards and you are familiar with the watercraft's safety guidelines. As an open water lifeguard, one of your responsibilities may be to patrol your zone using watercraft. Each facility will have its own rules and regulations regarding the use of watercraft, and you should make sure that you understand those that apply to you. As you patrol, check to see that the edges of your zone are clearly marked so that the safety limits are obvious to watercraft operators and swimmers. Your facility may also post signs at strategic areas to warn swimmers and boaters of the "swimmers only" sections of water.

INFORMING GUESTS

Signage

Your facility should have signs posted to inform guests of all relevant rules and warnings. These rules and warnings should be specific to your waterfront area and located in clearly visible locations (**Figure 14.6**). You may need to call a guest's attention to a particular sign or warning as you caution him or her regarding hazardous behavior. If a guest appears unable to understand or refuses to heed a warning sign, inform your supervisor immediately.

Flags

Flags are commonly used to alert swimmers of current water and weather conditions. Flags should be placed in a central location (**Figure 14.7**) along with an explanation of the meaning of each flag (**Figure 14.8**). Lifeguards or supervisors monitor the water and weather conditions and direct the placement of the correct flag.

A sample **flag system** may be:

- *Yellow*—The beach is open, and the water and weather conditions are safe for swimming.

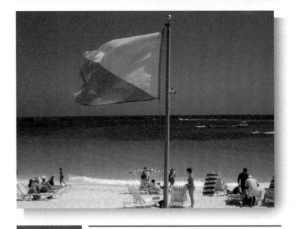

FIG 14.7　Flags can be used to indicate dangerous conditions.

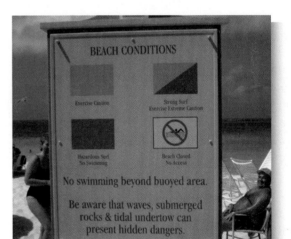

FIG 14.8　Flag explanations should be clearly posted.

- *Red and yellow*—Swimmers should use caution because weather and water conditions are changing and are being monitored.
- *Red*—The beach is closed due to dangerous water conditions and swimmers should not enter the water.

RESCUE EQUIPMENT

Open water lifeguards use much of the same equipment that pool lifeguards use. Additional specialized equipment may include:

- Binoculars
- Searching devices (e.g., masks, fins, snorkels, drag nets)

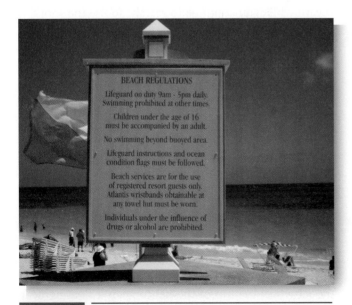

FIG 14.6　Signs should be posted to inform guests of all relevant rules and warnings.

- Scuba equipment
- Rescue boards and kayaks

Equipment must be reliable and easily accessible in an emergency. If equipment has been damaged, lost, or stolen, notify your supervisor immediately. Lifeguards need to know how to use all equipment at their facility. If there is some equipment you are unfamiliar with, let your supervisor know that you need instruction in its use.

Binoculars

Binoculars are standard equipment in larger open water environments. They make it possible for life-guards to recognize problems from a distance.

Searching Devices

Masks, fins, snorkels, and drag nets can be helpful for searching the bottom of the swimming area during facility inspections and guest-recovery situations (**Figure 14.9**). As with other equipment, you must become proficient in their use before you are involved in a rescue situation.

Masks

Masks assist you with seeing more clearly underwater and will protect your eyes. Masks are generally made from a flexible material that conforms to the user's face to keep water from entering. They come in various sizes and should have a safety glass viewing pane and a head strap that allows for quick, easy adjustment. To test the fit, place the mask over your face without securing the head straps and take a breath in through the nose creating suction to hold the mask in place. Water should not leak into the mask when your head is under the water. When the proper size mask is verified, place the head straps on and securely tighten them, being careful not to over tighten. If fogging of the mask is an issue, rub a small amount of saliva on the inside of the viewing pane and rinse.

Fins

Fins allow you to reach the guest more quickly and reduce the fatigue factor. They make it easier to tow a guest in distress back to shore and assist the lifeguard in lifting themselves out of the water to administer in-water breaths.

If you are using fins, they should be carried in one hand into the water until you reach mid-thigh or waist

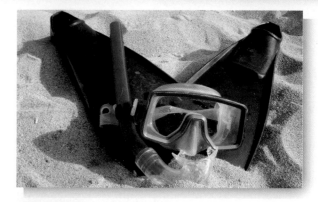

FIG 14.9   Mask, fins, and snorkel.

depth. You should then angle yourself sideways to the oncoming waves in order to put your fins on. Put them on one at a time, ensuring that you hold on tightly to the second fin as you put the first one on. Put your foot into the fin all the way and slide the strap over your heel. Be careful not to use the straps to pull the fins on as they may tear. If a dock or pier is available, fins may be put on prior to entering the water.

Snorkel

Snorkels allow you to breathe through a tube that extends above the surface of the water while keeping your face in the water and maintaining eye contact with the area beneath you. Snorkels are also designed to allow you to dive below the water, resurface, and quickly clear the water from the tube so that you may breath while you continue to search. To use the snorkel, breathe deeply and slowly through your mouth. When you want to submerge, take a deep breath, hold it, and dive below the surface. When you resurface, forcefully exhale to clear the water from the snorkel.

Drag Nets

Drag nets allow you to search a large area for a sub-merged guest in water that is less than chest deep. Drag nets can be made from a durable volleyball net or other suitable netting. They should be designed to stretch out to the desired width spanning a Zone of Protection area (or part of a zone). They should not be too large to be effectively used by two lifeguards. Poles should be attached to each end of the net so that it can be han-dled by the lifeguards; buoys should be attached along the length of the top of the net to keep it floating near the surface when in use. The bottom of the net should be weighted to keep it at the bottom. The net should be stored in an easily accessible location near the waterfront and it should be stored in a folded manner rather than rolled up, so it can be easily undone with minimal tangling in the event of an emergency.

Scuba Equipment

You may sometimes need scuba equipment to search the bottom of a swimming area if visibility is poor and the water is deep. Scuba diving involves a special training course, and rescue diving is even more specialized. Just because you are a scuba diver does not mean you are qualified to dive in a rescue situation in zero visibility water. Your supervisor will establish written policies and procedures for the use of scuba diving equipment and authorized personnel.

Rescue Boards and Kayaks

Many open water facilities use rescue boards or kayaks to help lifeguards reach distressed swimmers more quickly (**Figure 14.10**). Lifeguards may also be stationed on the rescue board/kayak at the perimeter of a swimming area during times when the facility is crowded. As an open water lifeguard, you must not use a rescue board or kayak unless you have received the necessary training.

≈≈ OPEN WATER RESCUES

When you are lifeguarding at an open water facility and you observe a swimmer in distress, begin your rescue attempt by blowing one loud, long blast of your whistle and raising a clenched fist to summon help. Then, carefully climb down from the lifeguard stand, taking all necessary equipment with you. Evacuate guests from the swimming area until another lifeguard is available to cover your zone—only attempt a rescue alone if no assistance is immediately available.

Getting Through the Surf

Whenever a lifeguard identifies a guest in distress, response time in reaching the guest is extremely important. Getting through the water and/or negotiating surf requires good fitness, speed, and technique. Once you start running into the shallow surf a **high knee action** is recommended (**Figure 14.11**), which will enable you to run further at a quicker rate. Once you reach mid-thigh or waist deep water, you should release your rescue tube and let it trail behind you and begin swimming or **dolphin diving** (see below).

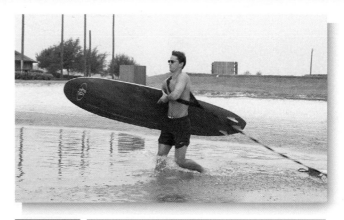

FIG 14.10 Rescue boards are used at many open water facilities.

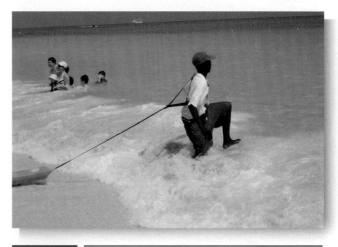

FIG 14.11 High knee action when running into a shallow surf.

Dolphin Diving

Release your rescue tube so that it is trailing behind you, and dive forward under the water/wave (**Figure 14.12**). Use the glide of the dive to make headway, resurface, and dive forward again. Time your dive so that it takes you underneath oncoming waves which will avoid you being dragged back towards the shore. This may be done several times before you reach a point where the water depth prevents you from diving forward any more. At this point you should begin to swim.

In big surf, it is important to be aware of breaking waves. It may be helpful to use a water polo swim style, where the head is upright for 2–3 strokes to observe any oncoming waves and ensure that you are heading in the right direction.

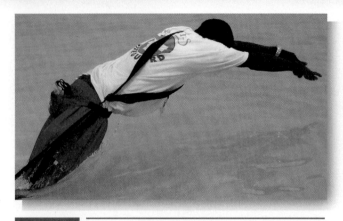

FIG 14.12 Position for dolphin diving.

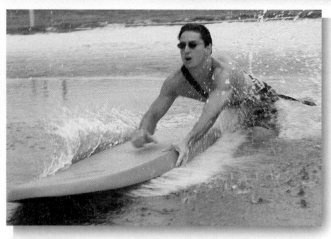

FIG 14.14 Mount the rescue board when you reach waist-deep water.

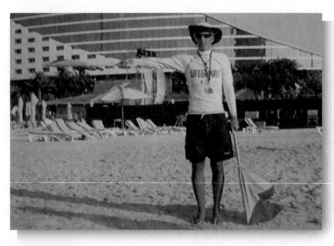

FIG 14.13 Communicating with hand signals and flags.

BEACH TO WATER COMMUNICATIONS

If the surf is rough or if the distressed swimmer submerges, the responding lifeguard may lose sight of the distressed swimmer. It is therefore a good idea to develop a set of signals that can be used to assist the in-water lifeguard by communicating from the beach to the water. These can be hand signals or small flags (**Figure 14.13**).

USING WATERCRAFT

If you are using a rescue board or kayak, you should be aware of any conditions that will enable you to make the best decision about where to enter the water. On a calm day, it would be best to enter the water with the rescue board or kayak by the most direct route and approach the swimmer from the water. In some circumstances, such as rip tides or currents, conditions can be used to assist the rescuer. For example, finding and moving toward a fast-moving current can assist the rescuer in getting out to sea and reduce the need to break through waves.

Once in the water, your rescue tube strap should be worn over the shoulder with the rescue tube trailing behind you as you make your way to the guest. When you reach an appropriate depth of water (waist deep for a rescue board and knee deep for a kayak) mount the board or kayak in the most suitable position and begin paddling towards the guest (**Figure 14.14**). On a rescue board, you can be in either a prone or a kneeling position, though the prone position gives greater stability because it maintains a lower center of gravity. Paddling on a rescue board is done either with the hands, using a butterfly or front crawl stroke, or using paddles (**Figure 14.15**). In a kayak, you will be in a seated or kneeling position, depending on the style of kayak, and will use paddles.

It is critical to practice your initial entry and mounting in order to master the balance required. When approaching the guest, approach from the side, collect your rescue tube, and dismount from the board or kayak.

RESCUE AND EXTRICATION

Gain control of the rescue tube before executing the appropriate rescue bringing the guest back to safety. If the guest is unconscious and not breathing, begin

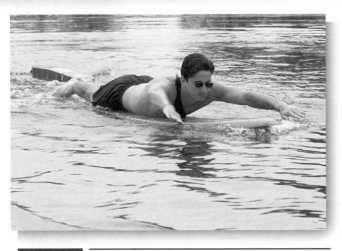

FIG 14.15   Paddling to the guest.

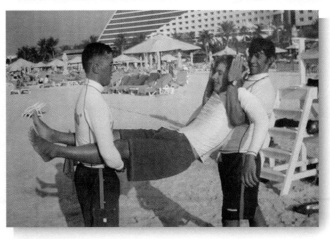

FIG 14.16   Carrying a guest.

rescue breathing while moving back toward the shore. If prevailing conditions make it impossible to provide rescue breathing in the water, then immediate extrication of the distressed swimmer must become the priority so that care can be administered as soon as possible. Assistance in getting back to shore can be provided by a second lifeguard who can extend his or her rescue tube as an additional aid and use it to tow you and the guest by either swimming or using the recovered rescue board or kayak. Once reaching shallow water, one or two rescuers should carry the guest from the water to a point on the beach where he or she can be assessed.

Carrying the Guest

Secure the guest under the armpits while maintaining an open airway. The higher you hold the guest, the easier it will be to drag him or her. Keep your back as straight as possible while dragging the guest to a safe point on the beach. If a second lifeguard is available, he or she can lift the guest's legs by placing both arms behind the knees, and both guards can carry the guest onto the beach (**Figure 14.16**). Slowly and gently lower the guest onto his or her back, ensuring that the head is constantly supported and an open airway is maintained.

MISSING PERSON SEARCH

If you suspect that a missing guest is submerged, the swimming area should be evacuated immediately. The technique used to conduct a missing guest search should be stated as part of the facility's EAP. The goal is to find, retrieve, and begin administering care to a submerged swimmer as quickly as possible within the 3-minute standard. Search techniques should be practiced and no person should be involved in a search unless he or she has been trained in the search techniques used at your facility.

There are two main techniques used in missing person searches: snorkel swim and net drag search.

Mask, Fin, and Snorkel Swim Search

In deep water, rescue teams will use the **mask, fin, and snorkel swim search**. Each member of the team will be equipped with mask, fins, and snorkel and will perform a coordinated series of surface dives. The search begins by forming a straight line at a point near where the submerged guest was last seen, keeping the guest's last known position in front of and in the center of the line. The line should extend to either side of the guest's last known position. If the guest's position/location is unknown, the line should form at the end of the Zone of Protection area, in to which the current is directed. Each lifeguard should be an arm's reach away from the next. As a group, guards should perform a surface dive to the bottom and swim a predetermined number of strokes in a straight line forward while keeping their hands in front of them in a sweeping motion. When all of the lifeguards surface, the group should move back a few feet, realign themselves, and repeat the process until the entire bottom has been searched or the missing guest has been located. Depending on the size of the zone and the number of lifeguards available, it may be necessary for the line to shift positions to move to the next area of

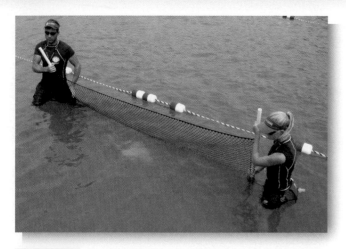

FIG 14.17 Net drag search.

the zone to be searched. This move should follow the direction of the current if the position where the guest submerged is known. If the guest's position is not known, the entire zone will need to be searched. It is crucial that the surface dives are coordinated to ensure that all areas are searched.

Net Drag Search

In shallow water, the **net drag search** technique can be used (**Figure 14.17**). When a net drag is needed for a missing person search, lifeguards must know their individual responsibilities. When the emergency response begins, two or more rescuers should retrieve the net and make their way to one end of the zone. The net is opened spanning the width of the zone and kept pulled tight to prevent a guest in distress being missed by the search net. Rescuers then walk the net along the length of the zone ensuring that the bottom of the net drags along the water's bottom. All rescuers continually scan the general area surrounding them. Be sure to communicate and not miss any areas.

As with the mask, fin, and snorkel swim search, it may be necessary to realign drag net to cover the entire part of the zone that is to be searched (**Figure 14.18**). When realigning, the guard who is on the end in the direction the net is to move should remain stationary and act as a pivot point. This will allow the guard at the other end of the net to move around him/her, ensuring that there is no gap between drags once the move has been made. This process should be repeated until the entire area has been searched or the guest has been located.

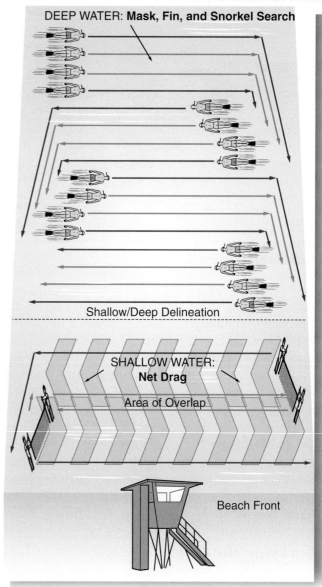

FIG 14.18 The mask, fin, and snorkel swim search and the net drag search.

〰️ PUTTING IT ALL TOGETHER

When a guest goes missing, time is critical. Many factors will impact your ability to recover the missing person within the confines of the 10/3 protection standard. The larger the Zone of Protection area, the longer it will take for a bottom search to be completed. The number of available lifeguards will also greatly affect this process. The more lifeguards available or the smaller the Zone of Protection area; the less time the search will take.

To be effective at maintaining the 10/3 protection standard, it is imperative that each facility have a documented procedure for conducting a missing person search as part of their EAP. The procedures must take minimum staffing levels and the size of the zones to be searched into account. When possible net drag searches and mask, fin, and snorkel swim searches should be done simultaneously by two teams of lifeguards. For single guarded facilities, or facilities with only a few lifeguards on duty, this may not be possible. In these cases proper planning and education will enable the guards to organize themselves to quickly and efficiently complete a bottom search using these techniques.

The key to successful implementation of search techniques is to know and understand the facility's EAP, and to regularly practice search and rescue techniques utilizing all of the necessary equipment.

WRAP-UP

Being a professional open water lifeguard involves:

- Understanding the differences between pool and open water lifeguarding

- Knowing the common causes of incidents at open water facilities

- Being aware of how environmental changes can impact open water facilities

- Being able to perform an open water rescue

- Maintaining your skill level through practice with equipment used at your facility

WHAT YOU SHOULD HAVE LEARNED

After reading this chapter and completing the related course work, you should be able to:

1. Describe how surveillance techniques of an open water facility differ from those of a pool.

2. Describe how the equipment used for open water lifeguarding differs from pool lifeguarding.

3. Demonstrate how to use watercraft to assist with a rescue.

4. Describe how to perform an open water rescue.

CHAPTER 14 *Lifeguard Skills*

OPEN WATER LIFEGUARDING

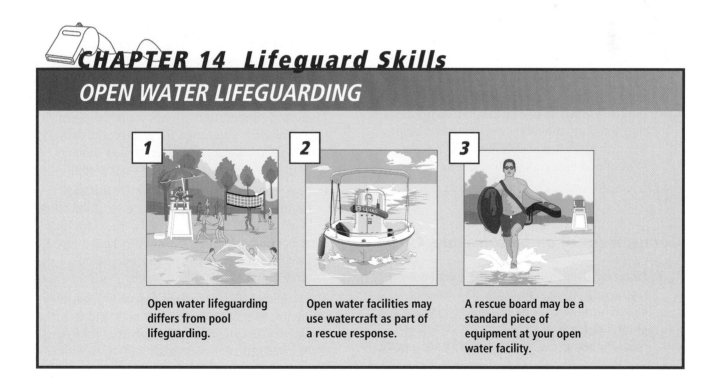

1 Open water lifeguarding differs from pool lifeguarding.

2 Open water facilities may use watercraft as part of a rescue response.

3 A rescue board may be a standard piece of equipment at your open water facility.

Appendix A
Sample Emergency Action Plans (EAPs)

In these EAPs, the rescue team consists of a rescuing lifeguard, an off-duty lifeguard, and a supplemental responder. Supplemental responders are non-lifeguard responders trained in deck extrication for unconscious guests and/or guests with suspected neck or back injury, cardiopulmonary resuscitation (CPR), foreign body airway obstruction (FBAO), automated external defibrillator (AED) use, and supplemental oxygen support (SOS) systems.

～～～ SINGLE LIFEGUARD EAP

On-duty lifeguard identifies and recognizes a distressed guest and initiates the EAP by giving one long whistle blast. Lifeguard then enters water and executes the appropriate rescue (see below).

Management of an Active (Responsive) Guest

1. Off-duty lifeguard provides backup coverage of the rescuing lifeguard's zone until the lifeguard returns to the stand.
2. Rescuing lifeguard completes the rescue, assists the guest from the pool/attraction, completes a rescue report, and follows up on causal factors (e.g., inexperienced swimmer in deep water who should be wearing a lifejacket).
3. Lifeguard rotates back into position.

Management of an Unconscious Guest

1. Rescuing lifeguard positions the guest on a rescue tube, opens the airway, and assesses breathing while moving toward the extrication point. Lifeguard calls out for a backboard and medical/trauma bag to arrive at extrication point.

2. If guest is not breathing, lifeguard performs rescue breathing with a resuscitation mask while moving toward the extrication point.
   a. Simultaneously, the off-duty lifeguard communicates to a supplemental responder (and/or communication central) for assistance. This guard should then clear the pool/attraction, facilitate bringing the backboard to the extrication point, and communicate with the primary lifeguard.
   b. Simultaneously, the supplemental responder (and/or communication central) will call 9-1-1 or use other means of EMS communication for assistance. This guard should then bring the trauma bag and AED to the pool/attraction, prepare equipment for use, and prepare to assist with extrication if necessary.
3. Once extrication is achieved, the guest should be moved 6 feet from the water's edge and remain on the backboard.
4. The rescue team (lifeguard, off-duty lifeguard, and responder) will assess the guest and provide care as needed (e.g., CPR, AR, FBAO, AED, SOS).
5. If AED is needed, one rescuer will prepare the guest for application of pads while the other two rescuers continue CPR and oxygen delivery, facilitated with the use of an oxygen adapter until AED application has been completed.
6. Continue care until EMS arrives or the guest begins to breathe on his or her own. If the guest begins breathing on his or her own, place him or her in the recovery position and continue to provide supplemental oxygen with a non-rebreathing mask.
7. Complete incident reports and collect witness names, addresses, phone numbers, and factual witness statements. Do not begin an interview or investigative process with staff or witnesses.

Management of a Guest with Suspected Neck and Back Injury

1. Rescuing lifeguard performs an ease-in entry, calls for backboard, and executes spinal management skills to secure inline stabilization.

   a. Simultaneously, the off-duty lifeguard communicates to a supplemental responder (and/or communication central) to complete 9-1-1 or other means of EMS communication, clears pool of other guests, and brings the backboard to the pool/attraction.

   b. Simultaneously, the supplemental responder should bring the trauma bag and AED to the pool/attraction and assist with clearing guests and/or backboarding procedures if more than two guards are required.

2. If the two-lifeguard backboarding procedure is in place, the rescuing lifeguard and off-duty lifeguard will work as a team to facilitate proper strapping and head immobilization of the guest.

3. Lifeguards should perform proper and safe extrication and continue with assessment and care until EMS personnel arrive.

4. Complete incident reports and collect witness names, addresses, phone numbers and factual witness statements. Do not begin an interview or investigative process with staff or witnesses.

MULTIPLE LIFEGUARD EAP

On-duty lifeguard identifies and recognizes a distressed guest and initiates the EAP by giving one long whistle blast. Lifeguard then enters water and executes the appropriate rescue (see below).

Management of an Active (Responsive) Guest

1. Designated lifeguard provides backup coverage of the rescuing lifeguard's zone until the lifeguard returns to the stand.

2. Rescuing lifeguard completes rescue and assists the guest from the pool/attraction.

3. Manager, supervisor, or lead will complete a rescue report and follow up on causal factors (e.g., inexperienced swimmer in deep water who should be wearing a lifejacket).

4. Lifeguard rotates back into position.

Management of an Unconscious Guest

1. Rescuing lifeguard positions the guest on a rescue tube, opens the airway, and assesses breathing while moving toward the extrication point. Lifeguard calls out for a backboard to arrive at extrication point.

2. If guest is not breathing, lifeguard performs rescue breathing with a resuscitation mask while moving toward the extrication point.

3. Manager, supervisor, or lead will continue the communication process (site-specific details) both internally (for additional levels of response and equipment facilitation of trauma bag, including SOS and AED) and externally (to contact EMS).

4. Manager, supervisor, or lead will bring the backboard to the pool/attraction and communicate with the rescuing lifeguard to move to the extrication point.

5. Additional levels of response (supervisors, leads, EMS personnel) will bring the trauma bag and AED to the pool/attraction, glove up, and prepare equipment for use as the lifeguards extricate the guest.

6. Once extrication is achieved, the guest should be moved 6 feet from the water's edge and remain on the backboard.

7. The rescue team (rescuing lifeguard and manager, supervisor, lead, and/or EMS personnel) will assess the guest and provide care as needed.

8. Continue providing care until EMS arrives or the guest begins to breathe on his or her own. If the guest begins breathing on his or her own, place him or her in the recovery position and continue providing supplemental oxygen with a non-rebreathing mask. Patient may continue to require additional care.

9. Complete incident reports and collect witness names, addresses, phone numbers, and factual witness statements. Do not begin an interview or investigative process with staff or witnesses.

Management of a Guest with Suspected Neck and Back Injury

1. Rescuing lifeguard performs an ease-in entry, calls for backboard, and executes spinal management skills to secure inline stabilization.

2. Manager, supervisor, or lead will continue the communication process (site-specific details) both internally (for additional levels of response and equipment facilitation of backboard) and externally (to contact EMS).

3. Manager, supervisor, or lead will bring the backboard to the pool/attraction and work as a team to complete proper strapping and head immobilization of guest.

4. Lifeguards should perform proper and safe extrication and continue with assessment and care until EMS personnel arrive.

5. Complete incident reports and collect witness names, addresses, phone numbers, and factual witness statements. Do not begin an interview or investigative process with staff or witnesses.

Appendix B
Sample Rescue Flow Charts

≈≈≈ UNCONSCIOUS GUEST

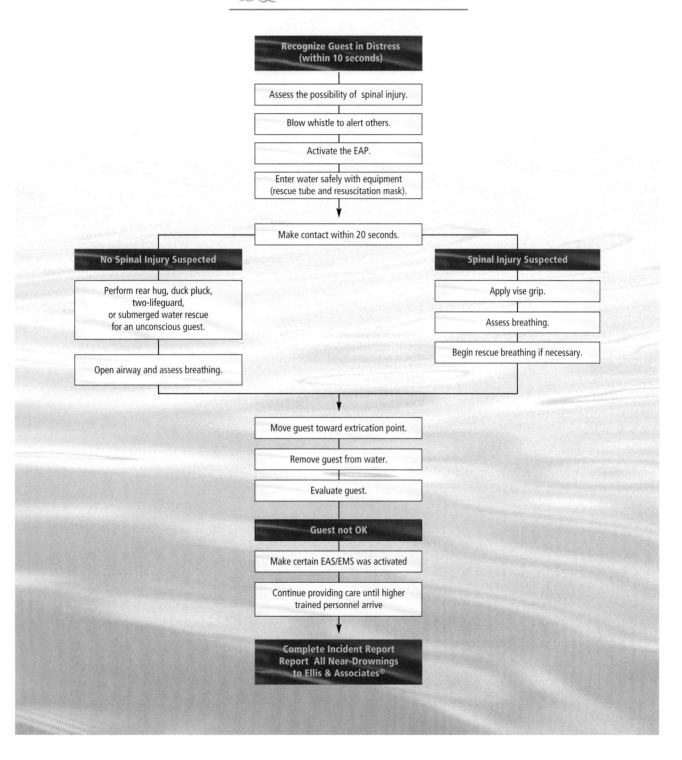

Recognize Guest in Distress (within 10 seconds)

Assess the possibility of spinal injury.

Blow whistle to alert others.

Activate the EAP.

Enter water safely with equipment (rescue tube and resuscitation mask).

Make contact within 20 seconds.

No Spinal Injury Suspected

Perform rear hug, duck pluck, two-lifeguard, or submerged water rescue for an unconscious guest.

Open airway and assess breathing.

Spinal Injury Suspected

Apply vise grip.

Assess breathing.

Begin rescue breathing if necessary.

Move guest toward extrication point.

Remove guest from water.

Evaluate guest.

Guest not OK

Make certain EAS/EMS was activated

Continue providing care until higher trained personnel arrive

Complete Incident Report Report All Near-Drownings to Ellis & Associates®

CONSCIOUS GUEST

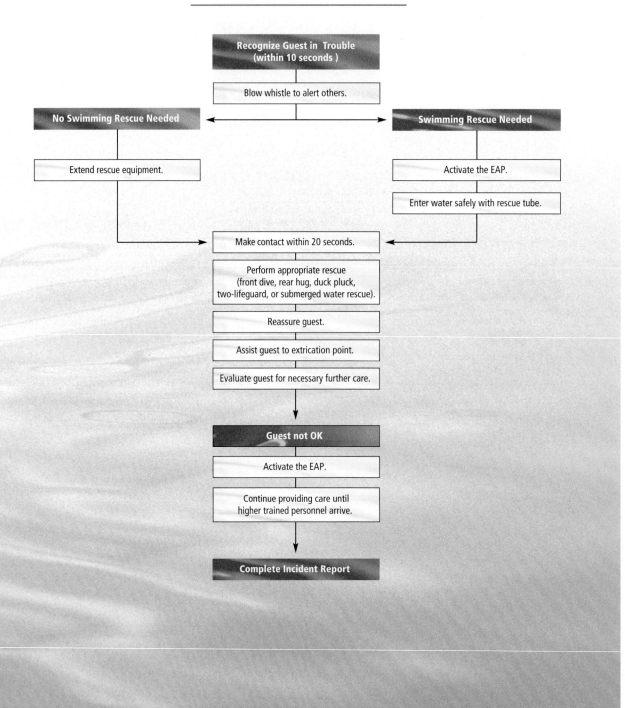

Recognize Guest in Trouble (within 10 seconds)

Blow whistle to alert others.

No Swimming Rescue Needed — **Swimming Rescue Needed**

Extend rescue equipment.

Activate the EAP.

Enter water safely with rescue tube.

Make contact within 20 seconds.

Perform appropriate rescue (front dive, rear hug, duck pluck, two-lifeguard, or submerged water rescue).

Reassure guest.

Assist guest to extrication point.

Evaluate guest for necessary further care.

Guest not OK

Activate the EAP.

Continue providing care until higher trained personnel arrive.

Complete Incident Report

Glossary of Key Terms

10/3 protection standard—Practice that requires a lifeguard to visually scan the Zone of Protection area every 10 seconds, identifying any distressed guests. The lifeguard then has 3 minutes to perform the proper rescue and begin rendering aid.

10/20 protection standard—Practice that requires a lifeguard to visually scan the Zone of Protection area every 10 seconds, identifying any distressed guests. The lifeguard then has 20 seconds to reach the guest and begin rendering aid.

Abdominal thrust—Upward pushing motion on the abdomen to remove a foreign body obstruction and open the airway.

Abrasion—Superficial skin damage caused by a scrape.

Active drowning—Drowning in which the guest struggles on the surface for a short period before submerging.

Agonal breaths—Occasional gasping breaths that often occur when the heart stops beating in cases of cardiac arrest.

Approach stroke—Any combination of leg kicks and arm movements that allow the lifeguard to make the fastest forward progress in the water.

Assist—Action of helping a distressed swimmer while being able to maintain the 10/20 protection standard in the Zone of Protection area.

Audit—Process through which lifeguards are held accountable for maintaining their skills and professionalism at "test-ready" standards at all times. It is designed to identify potential risk exposures before they become catastrophic.

Automated external defibrillator (AED)—Device that analyzes the heart's rhythm and signals the need to administer an electric shock (defibrillation) to a patient in cardiac arrest.

Backboard—Rigid board with straps that secure the body and a device that secures the head. It is used to remove a guest with a suspected spinal injury from the water while minimizing the movement of the body and the head or to assist in extricating an unconscious guest from the water.

Backboarding—Process used by two or more lifeguards to remove a guest with a suspected spinal cord injury from the water without further injury to the spinal column.

Bag valve mask (BVM)—Device consisting of a face mask attached to a bag with a reservoir and connected to oxygen; capable of delivering 90 percent supplemental oxygen to a guest.

Body substance isolation (BSI)—Protective devices and measures taken by rescuers to limit or eliminate direct contact with blood or potentially infectious bodily fluids.

Cardiac arrest—Point in time when the heart has stopped pumping blood and is no longer functioning.

Cardiopulmonary resuscitation (CPR)—A combination of chest compressions and rescue breathing used to help deliver oxygen to the brain via the lungs until EMS arrives. It is used for someone who is not breathing and does not have a pulse.

Compact jump—Entry into the water from a height. The lifeguard keeps the rescue tube up under the armpits, feet flat, and knees slightly bent. It is designed to minimize the risk of injury to the lifeguard while allowing for speed in initiating a rescue.

Crowd control—Giving directions to or controlling the behavior of a large group of people at one time.

Deep water rescue—Rescue in which the guest in distress is submerged beyond arm's reach.

Defibrillation—Delivery of an electric shock to a patient in cardiac arrest, momentarily stopping all electrical activity in the heart and allowing the pacemaker cells to produce a coordinated heartbeat.

Dehydration—Loss of water in the body.

Distress—Condition in which a guest is unable to maintain a position on top of the water or make progress to safety without assistance.

Distressed swimmer rescue—Rescue for a guest who has shown an inability to remain upon or return to the surface of the water.

Dolphin diving—Rescue technique of moving through waves or water while wearing fins.

Drowning—Death caused by accumulation of a fluid in the lungs or a laryngospasm.

Dry drowning—Asphyxiation, or suffocation, resulting from a laryngospasm with no water present in the distressed guest's lungs.

Duck pluck rescue—Technique in which the lifeguard reaches over the rescue tube and below the surface of the water to grasp a submerged guest within reach.

Emergency action plan (EAP)—Written plan for a specific facility outlining step-by-step emergency procedures and responsibilities.

Emergency medical services (EMS)—Trained personnel who respond to an emergency when 9-1-1 or a local emergency number is called.

Epiglottis—Cartilage behind the tongue that works like a valve over the windpipe.

Extension assist—Helping a guest reach safety by extending an arm or a rescue tube.

Eye avulsion—An injury in which the eye globe is completely removed from the skull.

Feet-first surface dive—Method of propelling the body toward the bottom, feet first, by pushing the water upward with the arms.

Flag system—System by which centrally located colored flags are used to alert guests and guards of changing weather conditions.

Foreign body—Object that causes an obstruction or blockage of the airway.

Front drive rescue—Rescue technique used when a guest is actively in distress on top of the water, performed with a rescue tube.

Golden Rule of guest relations—Treat people as you would like to be treated—with respect.

Guest relations—The way that you treat and respond to guests at your facility.

Head tilt with chin-lift—Method of opening the airway that entails tilting the head back while lifting the chin.

Heat cramps—Cramps in the muscles caused by loss of water and salt from the body due to overexposure to heat.

Heat emergencies—Emergencies that occur when a person spends too much time in a hot environment without taking in enough fluid to maintain the body's equilibrium.

Heat exhaustion—Heat-related illness that is caused by the loss of significant amounts of fluid from perspiration. Symptoms include profuse sweating, fatigue, nausea, vomiting, and cool, pale, sweaty skin.

Heat stroke—Life-threatening condition in which the body temperature rises due to overexposure to heat and breakdown of the body's temperature control system.

Heimlich maneuver—Technique of clearing a nonbreathing patient's blocked airway by providing abdominal thrusts.

High knee action—Rescue technique of moving through shallow surf at a quick pace.

High risk—Conditions or characteristics that make it more likely for an accident or incident to happen.

Hyperglycemia—Condition in which a diabetic has too much blood sugar.

Hypoglycemia—Condition in which a diabetic has too little blood sugar.

Hypothermia—Medical condition in which the body loses heat.

Hypoxic convulsions—Condition that occurs due to a lack of oxygen in the brain. It may cause a person to appear rigid or stiff, jerk violently, and/or froth at the mouth.

Inline stabilization—Maintaining head and neck alignment with the torso, for guests with suspected spinal injury.

In-service training—Ongoing training received after obtaining lifeguard certification and becoming employed at an aquatic facility.

Intervertebral discs—Circular cushions of cartilage that separate the vertebrae in the spine.

Jaw-thrust with head tilt—Method of opening the airway in guests without suspected spinal injury.

Jaw-thrust without head tilt—Method of opening the airway in guests with suspected spinal injury.

Laryngospasm—Condition in which water droplets irritate the epiglottis, causing it to close over the glottis and preventing air from entering the air passage.

Liability—Legal responsibility.

Life-threatening—Quality of an injury or condition that could cause loss of life if specific care is not given.

Mask, fin, and snorkel swim search—Search performed when a guest is submerged in deep water, coordinated by a rescue team performing surface dives.

Mechanism of injury—Means by which an incident occurred. This information should be gathered by the first responder for the incident report and provided to EMS personnel.

Net drag search—Rescue technique involving a drag net, poles, and buoys to search a specified area of open water.

Overarm vise grip—Method of stabilizing a guest with suspected spinal injury who is face up in the water.

Passive (silent) drowning—Drowning caused by various physical conditions, such as heart attack or stroke, in which the guest shows no signs of struggle at the surface of the water.

Primary check—Examining or checking a person for any life-threatening condition.

Professional image—Impression of responsibility, authority, friendliness, and competency. It is demonstrated by the way lifeguards look and act toward guests.

Pulse—Verification of a beating heart.

Rapid extrication—Removal of a nonbreathing guest, who is not suspected of having a spinal cord injury, from the water.

Rear hug rescue—Technique used for a guest who is on the surface of the water facing away from the rescuer. It can be used on an unconscious or conscious guest and is always performed with a rescue tube.

Recovery position—Position in which a guest is on his or her side so gravity will aid in moving the tongue away from the back of the throat and allow for the passage of air and drainage of fluids.

Rescue—Situation in which a lifeguard enters the water to aid a guest in distress.

Rescue breathing—Method of providing oxygen from a rescuer to a guest who is not breathing but has a pulse.

Rescue tube—Piece of rescue equipment with a strap and line made of vinyl-dipped foam for buoyancy.

Respiratory arrest—Sudden stoppage of breathing.

Resuscitation mask—Barrier device that provides protection from infectious diseases to the rescuer while he or she is providing rescue breathing or CPR.

Risk management—Reducing the likelihood of an accident by controlling the factors that make the situation high risk.

Rotation—System employed each time a lifeguard leaves his or her post and is relieved by another lifeguard.

Scanning—Moving the eyes and head throughout the top, middle, and bottom sections of a Zone of Protection area while maintaining the 10/20 or 10/3 protection standard.

Seizure—Sudden involuntary changes in the activity level of brain cells, usually due to disease, trauma, overdose, or chemical reactions.

Shock—Collapse of circulatory function caused by severe injury, blood loss, or disease.

Spinal cord—Group of nerve tissues that carries messages from the brain to the rest of the body and passes through the center of the spinal column.

Spinal injury—Injury to the spinal cord, usually caused by a blow to the head, neck, or spine. Compression or severing of the spinal cord can cause paralysis or death.

Spine—Column of 33 vertebrae that extend from the base of the head to the tip of the tailbone.

Splint—A flexible or rigid appliance used to protect and maintain the position of an injured extremity.

Squeeze play—Technique similar to the vise grip, used to stabilize a standing or sitting guest who is displaying the signs and symptoms of a spinal injury.

Standard of care—Expected level of skills and care at which lifeguards are expected to perform.

Submersion event—Incident in which a guest submerges beneath the surface of the water and will become a drowning victim if not rescued.

Submersion incident rescue—Rescue for a guest who is rendered unconscious and submerges under the surface of the water.

Supplemental responder—Non-lifeguard staff members trained to provide rescue and patient care skills as part of the lifeguard team in accordance with a facility's emergency action plan (EAP).

Two-lifeguard rescue—Process of two lifeguards working together, combining the front drive and the rear hug to "sandwich" a guest.

Underarm vise grip—Method of stabilizing a guest with suspected spinal injury who is face down in the water.

Ventricular fibrillation—Life-threatening rapid and disorganized heart rhythm; the most common cause of sudden and unexpected cardiac arrest in adults.

Ventricular tachycardia—Abnormal heart rhythm that causes the heart to beat too fast to effectively pump blood.

Vertebrae—Bones and segments composing the spinal column.

Vise grip—Rescue technique used to prevent further injury to a guest who is suspected of having suffered a spinal injury.

Wet drowning—Drowning caused by fluid accumulation in the lungs.

Zone of Protection—Area for which a lifeguard is responsible for scanning and maintaining the 10/20 or 10/3 protection standard.

Index